PATIENT 1

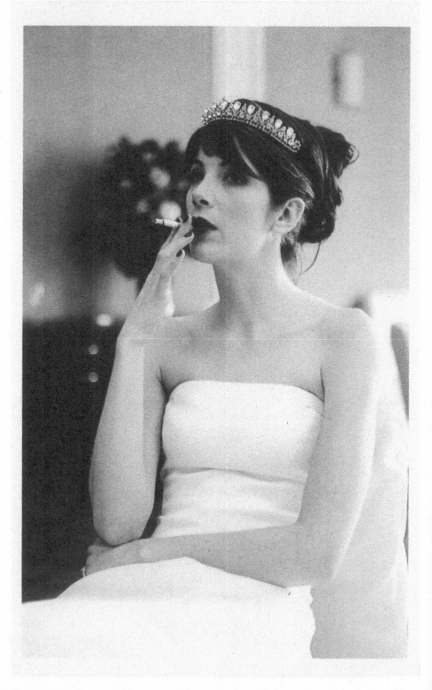

The smoking bride

PATIENT 1

Forgetting and Finding Myself

Charlotte Raven

with Daniel Raven

with an Afterword
by Professor Ed Wild

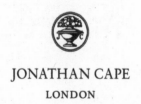

JONATHAN CAPE

LONDON

1 3 5 7 9 10 8 6 4 2

Jonathan Cape is part of the Penguin Random House group of companies whose addresses can be found at global.penguinrandomhouse.com.

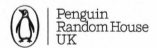

Copyright © Charlotte Raven 2021
Afterword © Ed Wild 2021

Charlotte Raven has asserted her right to be identified as the author of this Work in accordance with the Copyright, Designs and Patents Act 1988

First published by Jonathan Cape in 2021

penguin.co.uk/vintage

A CIP catalogue record for this book is available from the British Library

ISBN 9781787332331

Typeset in 11.5/16 pt Sabon LT Std
by Integra Software Services Pvt. Ltd, Pondicherry

Printed and bound in Great Britain by Clays Ltd, Elcograf S.p.A.

The authorised representative in the EEA is Penguin Random House Ireland, Morrison Chambers, 32 Nassau Street, Dublin D02 YH68.

Penguin Random House is committed to a sustainable future for our business, our readers and our planet. This book is made from Forest Stewardship Council® certified paper.

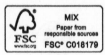

MIX
Paper from
responsible sources
FSC® C018179

To Anna and John

Introduction

This book started life as an autobiographical blog about living with Huntington's disease, a degenerative neurological condition that causes cognitive impairments, short- and long-term memory loss, changes in personality and a movement disorder called chorea. It is rare – only 6,000 people in the UK have it – so talking to medical professionals about it can be difficult, as they've often never heard of it.

I started writing the blog in 2017 as an awareness-raising exercise, and was pleased when people from the HD community who had never reached out to anyone before got in touch and trusted me with their stories. I sent the link to the Huntington's Disease Association, who asked if I'd mind them sharing it with doctors and specialist care agencies, and I got lots of positive feedback when they did. Some of them said they could tell I was a professional writer.

This was only half true, though. I had indeed been a successful newspaper columnist in the 90s and often found myself wishing I'd never given it up, but my history with longer form works was not a happy one. Conversations with my agent towards the tail end of my time as a columnist resulted in a book idea that seemed ambitious but achievable: a feminist conduct book about false consciousness addressed to an imaginary teenager. It was to be called *Advice to a Young Girl on Avoiding the Illusions of her Sex* – a title I *really* liked – and we found a publisher for it surprisingly quickly. I wanted to write a feminist classic that would be remembered and talked about for years after my death – so no pressure, then.

The publishers were patient and I met the editor every few months to check in with him. I kept saying I'd nearly finished but in fact I was just rewriting the first chapter over and over again. It took me ten years to realise that it wasn't working, by which time it had changed from a feminist advice book to a self-lacerating attack on my own narcissism. I shredded the 100-page manuscript and threw it in the bin, then deleted it from my computer so there would be no way back to it.

My children were shocked when I destroyed the book of doom in front of them but it felt good to me. When I eventually returned to my desk it was with a different perspective on writing, and more realistic expectations about what would be possible given my cognitive impairments and other difficulties. I felt like my story was backing up in my mind and I needed to find a form quickly; with HD attacking my memory, this really was the last chance saloon. A writer friend suggested I try writing a blog about the illness and its effects on the people around me, with some personal history woven in.

I called the blog *Forgetting Myself*, to reflect the fact that my identity was as imperilled as my cognitive processes. My carer helped me set it up and the friend who'd suggested it edited it, so it looked quite polished. I updated it every couple of weeks and felt more emboldened with every post.

I worried what my husband Tom would think about the way I was portraying him, as our marriage was in the process of breaking down and I was chronicling that as well as the intrusions of my illness. It was a difficult balancing act and I may not always have succeeded, as my ambivalence led to inconsistencies: I deified him one minute and deplored him the next, when neither view was entirely justified. Mostly, though, I realised that the evidence I'd amassed to indict him was outweighed by the case against me, and couldn't help feeling guilty about the way I'd behaved towards him before I got ill.

HD is an interesting illness so I was never short of material, and at least I didn't have any competitors – I was glad to be writing about a rare illness rather than, say, food or cats. But I soon started to feel like the posts were floating up into a cloud and never really landing anywhere, so in a cynical bid to give the public what they wanted I wrote about my deranged cat Archie, 'the Staffy of cats', who regularly attacked my carers and sometimes drew blood. I got more comments than I'd ever had for the posts about my own derangement.

When Tom finally saw the blog, he called me out for invading our children's privacy. But he was supportive of me and saw its potential to evolve into a book – as I was secretly starting to hope it would.

Although it had never exactly been what you'd call enjoyable, writing about my situation and trying to put the jigsaw-puzzle pieces of my life together on the page had felt therapeutic and even necessary. I wanted to extend this approach and bring in more stuff about my past while I could still remember it, but the blog clearly wasn't the right place for that. I wanted to write a book, but only if I could avoid the conventions of the standard misery memoir. I had many examples of this genre on my shelves but they were just for 'hate-reading' – I wasn't a fan. The authors all bragged about the journeys they'd been on but never really seemed to learn anything about themselves, and often ended up with bigger egos than when they'd started. For all their claims of searing honesty, they lacked self-awareness. If I didn't want to write something like that I'd need an angle on HD that felt fresh and true to my experience. The illness had challenged me and precipitated an existential crisis that I wanted to explore without constantly moaning about my symptoms.

I had become friends with Dr Ed Wild, a warm and approachable HD specialist who'd been there for me when the disease first sent my life spinning out of control, offering wise counsel on everything from barbiturates to my failing marriage. It occurred to me that if we worked on a book together, his medical account of the illness could complement my personal one. Ed said he was up for it and I was thrilled to have him on board; a joint enterprise felt much less daunting than a solo project.

We decided that the best way for me to approach my chapters would be to mix my recollections with updates on whatever was happening in my life at the time of writing, so that the end result would feel like a cross between an autobiography and a blog. It would be organised as a series of themed chapters, so the autobiographical elements wouldn't always be in chronological order, but the updates would.

This part of the plan rather alarmed me at first, as grouping my many and varied tribulations under neatly divided subject headings sounded like a much more challenging task than simply telling my story from A to Z, but then I realised that it made perfect sense: I had experienced HD as a dramatic, non-linear series of assaults, so any confusion in the book's chronology would mirror mine.

I finished the first three chapters in record time. But HD has made my consciousness chaotic and this is reflected in my writing – it is as untidy as my mind, which is as untidy as my bedroom. I am annoyed and I am annoying. I am inconsistent and unreliable. I wanted this book to be an accurate record of what it is like to exist with HD and to feel your brain and personality crumble. If it's exasperating to read this, imagine what it is like for me to live it. The way I express myself is a weird combination of my old voice and the authentic, disrupted voice of the illness, and I'm as likely to leave important stuff out as I am to include stuff that's extraneous. I needed a good editor, and someone who knew me well enough to fill in any gaps in my recall or rhetoric. I found both in the form of my brother, Dan, who knows me better than almost anyone.

I was halfway through writing the book in 2019 when Ed appeared on the news: there was a new HD drug that everyone was getting very excited about, and he was part of the team running the trial. I had known this for a while as he'd kept me in the loop during our conversations at the clinic, but it still felt miraculous. My blog meant that I was at the head of the queue to be asked for a quote and reaction to the breakthrough, and I was interviewed on Radio 4's *The World Tonight*. I hated talking on the radio but made myself do it. They asked why I'd taken the genetic test for HD, when I'd been diagnosed and what had happened to me since – these were all hard questions to put into soundbites, so I didn't do very well.

I knew it would make my story even more interesting if I turned out to be one of the participants in the trial – but that was out of my control, so I tried not to think about it. I had put my name down, along with lots of other people who deserved a place just as much as (if not more than) me, so now there was nothing to do but wait. And write.

I wrote and wrote, like my life depended on it – which I suppose it did, in a way – but I wasn't enjoying it. I'd always found writing difficult, but having HD makes it almost impossible. It's like driving a dodgy car whose MOT has expired; I do know what's wrong with it but that doesn't help, as there's no one around to fix it and I wouldn't have time to stop anyway. Writing a whole book under these conditions is like going on a motorway with no roadside assistance. I used to dread going into my study, turning on the computer and trying to find my place in the jumble of words on the screen.

A few weeks after I finished what I thought would be my last chapter, I found out that I *did* have a place on the trial. This changed everything: the most interesting (or at least newsworthy) part of the journey was now yet to come. I took extensive notes throughout the process and used those as the basis for a new final chapter.

When I was writing this book, I thought there were only two ways it could end: one where I was happy because I'd got on the trial and another where I was miserable because I hadn't, but still learned some life lessons from HD that weren't dependent on the new drug. I never imagined I'd end up getting both the trial and the lessons, but that's how it's turned out. Before I started the trial it seemed like the answer to all my problems, but then I realised it wasn't – I actually needed to change my mindset and learn to live with HD. The path was long and thorny but I think I got there in the end.

Ironically, I could never have written this book if I hadn't been intellectually compromised by my illness. It has humbled me and helped me connect more with the people around me, which is a newly acquired skill that I've been working on with commitment and persistence. No one has been 'roasted' – a hallmark of my previous work – and I feel like I've finally been able to portray my family and friends as they really are instead of as I'd like them to be. They are coming to life.

I

At Risk

The day I found out how I was going to die began innocuously enough: the usual blur of nappy changing and tetchy texts to my husband. Life in our recently refurbished house in Kentish Town had settled into a rhythm with a low level background of domestic discontent. Arguments about wallpaper had run their course, our two huge cats had made their peace with our daughter and I was pleased to have married a responsible hedonist who really liked babies but never made me feel guilty for finding them boring. My biggest worry was being a middle-class cliché adjudicating between different types of organic nappy cream.

Anna was one year old. My friends had been surprised when I became an advocate of active birth and attachment parenting. For reasons that are hard to retrieve, I gave birth with no pain relief in a birth pool in our sitting room. This terrifying experience had the opposite effect to the one intended: I felt lukewarm about the baby and annoyed that all our visitors seemed so obsessed with her. She slept in our bed with us for a while but I was worried about suffocating her. The Moses basket felt like a betrayal. It was all very confusing. When she was six months old I felt strong enough to write a piece about my maternal ambivalence for the *Guardian*'s Family section. I never dared return to the drop-in at the active birth centre after that, so we spent a lot of time watching CBeebies at home.

My husband, Tom, had gone to work early as it was the last day of his shoot. He was a documentary director who was filming a series about the London Underground. After a sleepless night, I was eating breakfast with Anna when the landline rang. It was my dad's old friend Eric, a steadfastly supportive American who had been keeping an eye on him ever since my mum died four years earlier. We were all worried because Murph (everyone called my dad Murph, for reasons that remain unclear) had been making some bad decisions and then digging in defiantly. He had lost a lot of money on risky investments and shacked up with a younger woman called Lottie.

Eric said there was something he thought I should know: Lottie was saying that Murph had been diagnosed with Huntington's disease. I couldn't believe it but Eric assured me that it was true.

I'd never heard of the condition and had no idea what it was. But there was an urgency about the way Eric passed on this information that was compelling. And the fact that Murph himself had not told me about it made the revelation somehow more shocking – even before I knew what it would mean.

So of course I did the one thing you should never do if you suspect that you or someone you love has an illness: I googled Huntingdon's ('Did you mean Huntington's?'). Wikipedia made it sound a bit like Alzheimer's and a bit like Parkinson's but worse than both. It was a degenerative neurological condition. I kept speed-reading the page but nothing was going in. There was a lot of detailed science with accompanying diagrams intended for the layperson but probably only decipherable by experts. It sounded terrible; poor Murph. Though it made sense of some of the things I'd noticed about Murph since my mother died. He was twitchy and fidgety, and there was a kind of hesitancy to his once-confident stride. Then there was a bit about genetics. In dry Wiki-speak, 'HD is inherited in an autosomal dominant fashion. The probability of each offspring inheriting an affected gene is 50 per cent'. All the things described that would happen to my dad might also happen to me or my brother, and if I had the gene then my children would be at risk too. Unlike Alzheimer's, HD typically manifests in mid-life, between the ages of thirty-five and forty-five. I was thirty-five.

The first visible sign of Huntington's disease is the chorea – jerky, uncontrollable, involuntary movements in all parts of the body. As parts of the brain degenerate, patients suffer severe cognitive problems: loss of memory, loss of judgement, loss of the capacity to organise oneself. Due to the loss of motor skills and the writhing contortions that afflict them, patients find walking difficult and are prone to injury from falls. They lose the capacity to swallow and sometimes die of malnutrition. Their personality is often affected, too. Reports of aggressive, compulsive and sexually inappropriate behaviour are common. Towards the end, families often see no other option than to have their suffering relatives institutionalised. There is currently no cure for Huntington's disease.

I called Tom. It was about half past eight in the morning and he was on his way to film at Edgware Road station. I was in tears as I explained what Eric had told me and what I had read. As usual he tried to calm me down, but for once his insistence that the internet was bound to be exaggerating the scale of the disaster was sadly misplaced. And then the phone went dead. He had arrived at Edgware Road just minutes after a bomb had been detonated on a train in the tunnel beneath. It was 7 July 2005, and for the rest of the day he was out of contact, caught up in the aftermath of the worst terror attack the capital had ever seen.

I turned on BBC News 24 and watched events unfold. I kept trying Tom's phone but it was going straight to voicemail. There was no one else to call. I didn't want to alarm my brother, Dan, as he is a sensitive soul. My mother, Susan, would have been reassuring in just the right register – you need your mother at these moments. We had been knocked off-course. I can't remember many of the details of the day, but I do know how it felt. There was a sense that our lives had darkened around the edges. I was confused about Murph – why hadn't he told me about his diagnosis himself? When Tom came back into range I was weeping with relief, but still unable to process the news that had blindsided us.

A couple of weeks later, at my suggestion, we met Murph without Lottie in neutral territory: a pub halfway between London and his home in Brighton. The Fox and Hounds was characterless with no distinguishing marks but they sold Harvey's beer, so it was a good place as far as Murph was concerned. In the car on the way down I found myself defending him: I was on Murph's side – to start with, at least.

He arrived late and was clearly in bad shape, shaking as he always did when he was stressed. I felt sorry for him but I also realised we were never going to get a straight answer out of him. I already felt let down.

Once we'd ordered drinks and found a table, I asked Murph why he hadn't told me that HD was in our family. Unexpectedly, he was annoyed with me for asking. He said it was a mild illness, which wasn't what I'd read on Wikipedia – was he lying or just in denial about what was happening? He also insisted that Lottie hadn't told Eric about his diagnosis, but when I asked, 'Then how did Eric know?', he didn't have an answer. He said he'd thought about telling me himself but hadn't wanted to upset me. It was an odd meeting: he was denying telling anyone but not denying having HD. And, strange to relate, he was angry with *me* for questioning his integrity. We left not really understanding what had just happened.

It was hard to tell how different my life would have been if he'd been brave enough to tell me about his diagnosis when he first got it, but at least I would have been empowered to make informed decisions instead of making them blindfolded. I felt that he should have told me before I got married to Tom or, if not then, before we had Anna. I'd had a right to know but he hadn't treated me like an adult, and that felt like a betrayal of trust.

He had not, at that point, mentioned that his mother Ida had also suffered from HD. This is the first of many muddles. I now know that Ida had Huntington's disease but am still not sure how cross to be with Murph for keeping that from me. What's certain is that, for years, he thought he didn't have it, so couldn't pass it on to me. His late-onset HD didn't develop until he was in his late fifties.

He first became symptomatic in 2001, after my mother died. The whole family had lost its bearings but Murph physically manifested what the rest of us were feeling: I can still see him stumbling down Park Avenue on an ill-advised trip to New York, and the oddly shaky signature he'd leave on bills at the restaurants we never really ate at there. We didn't know what was wrong with him. He looked like he'd lost contact with the earth, which seemed like a metaphor for being ungrounded by grief. There was so much going on then, we didn't pay much attention to it – and although his symptoms did worsen over time, it happened so gradually that we hardly noticed. Every so often, one of his friends would ask me if I'd noticed how much slower he was walking.

They were worried about Murph, but wouldn't have dreamed of asking him directly. He had time-tested strategies for deflecting personal enquiries with humour and wit. He was an enigma who never gave straight answers to questions he didn't like. His real name was Vivian! That used to sound weird whenever I heard it, and I never called him Dad. He was always Murph to me, but we never worked out where the nickname had come from because he'd say something different every time he was asked. And what could you say about his sense of humour? Mischievous? Dan prefers elliptical; he would set up running jokes that ran for years, and used to drive my mother mad by saying he was a better poet than Bob Dylan.

Murph had always been an unreliable narrator of his own life. We knew hardly anything about his upbringing, which seems strange now but didn't then. Even the close friends he'd met in seamy Earls Court in the 60s (where he lived after he'd been dishonorably discharged from either the RAF or the marines, no one remembers which) knew very little about his childhood, although I've heard that it was not uncommon for people to suppress their own histories in that era of self-invention.

The fact that Murph had no backstory may well have been part of his appeal. At the age of twenty-one, handsome and charismatic, he had seemed fully formed, and was a big hit with all the disreputables in the pickled egg pubs on the Earls Court Road. They lived in bedsits with overflowing ashtrays on every surface, like in Patrick Hamilton's *Hangover Square*. In spite of his undeclared political allegiance, my mother pursued him concertedly when she met him there. She had lived all over the place, as her stepfather was in the army, but by this time she was working as a personal assistant at the *Evening Standard* newspaper.

Susan was a duffel-coated Marxist and defender of Russia, which should have been a bar to her getting together with a man who hated being pigeonholed but was actually a bit more right wing than he claimed to be. They argued about Vietnam and Stalin but always good-naturedly, and I know he was proud of her. When she was arrested at a CND demo and sent to Holloway prison, he wrote to her every day, came to get her when she was released and never judged her (as she judged herself) for not sticking it out for the whole sentence. I wouldn't have known about any of this if Murph's friends hadn't told me – he didn't do anecdotes.

It might have been unreasonable to expect Murph to change the habits of a lifetime but I needed straight talking. Denial is common in HD, but it's more than just a coping mechanism – it also has a neurological component. So there's every chance that Murph sincerely believed there was nothing wrong with him in those first few years after Susan's death. But surely the actual diagnosis, when it came, should not have been kept from his children?

His way of making important decisions was to write a list of pros and cons. I could picture him frowning at a long list of cons, including the possible loss of my hard-won mental equilibrium; I'd had a breakdown in the 90s that had mystified him, but since meeting Tom I'd been on a more even keel. Murph may have worried that it would jeopardise my tenuous recovery to receive such awful news at the very moment when I seemed happier than I had in years. But thinking that didn't make me any less annoyed with him.

The next year was characterised by rising panic. My experience of being at risk of HD was an existential dread that separated me from the people around me. I was becoming morbidly preoccupied with my own mortality in my mid-thirties, when my friends were having second children and trying to fit date nights into their busy lives. They were very kind and tried to be supportive, but I envied them. It all seemed so unfair, and it was: my future was to be determined by the genetic equivalent of a coin-toss, with a normal life on one side and an awful death on the other. It might have been easier to conceive of it as a punishment from God, as I've heard they do in parts of South America where HD is prevalent in poorer communities. The randomness of it was destabilising. It felt like a crisis of faith, even though I was an atheist. Had I believed in God, I would have been very cross with him – as it was, my anger turned inwards.

I was more afraid of living with HD than dying from it. The illness impairs quickly but takes ages to dispatch you. Suffering is drawn out over years rather than months. I was worried that, unlike Murph, I'd be unhealthily absorbed by each new act of the neurodegenerative drama as it unfolded, logging every loss.

There was one big decision I needed to make that I felt ill equipped for, a devil/deep blue sea dilemma where the path to the future looked to be paved with thorns whichever route I took. In 1993, an international team of research scientists discovered the HD gene. This breakthrough was a mixed blessing for the HD community: for the first time it was possible to test for the gene, but they were still a long way from finding a cure or even an effective treatment. Some of the symptoms could be managed by drugs. When I found out that this test was available, I almost wished it wasn't. I felt tired just thinking about all the mental and emotional hurdles I would have to clear in order to arrive at a decision that was right for me.

Should I take the test? I am a pessimist, so I was doomed whatever I decided to do. If I didn't take the test, I would have spent the rest of my life assuming I had HD and paralysed with anxiety, waiting for symptoms to develop. If I took it and tested negative, that would have changed everything. The dark edges would have been banished. But was the chance that that would happen worth the risk that it wouldn't? The odds of my having the gene were 50/50, but in my head they felt more like 99/1. Dan said he would only want to get tested if there was some hope of a cure, which made sense for someone who wasn't interested in having children but not necessarily for me.

Although Dan had always been a worrier, he had a knack of burying his head in the sand whenever his worries threatened to overwhelm him. He'd had a bad time at our primary school in South London – not exactly bullied, but not befriended – which I hadn't noticed at the time. We still have a picture of him from his first day and he looks like a lamb to the slaughter. I should have been more supportive of him but I was too involved with my social life, even at that age. Now I found myself envying his easy way with denial – it was like a protective shield around him, whereas I was badly defended against all the worrying things that were happening to us.

My initial assumption was that most people in my position would choose to take the test, so I was surprised to learn that 95 per cent of them don't. However (there was always a however), a survey of people at risk of HD that was carried out before the predictive test existed found 50 to 70 per cent of them saying they would definitely be interested in taking one if it did – suggesting (to me, at least) that wanting to take the test was the rational response, avoiding it the cowardly cop-out.

Murph didn't want me to be tested. I started on a pros and cons list of my own without really trusting this method, which had always struck me as a failure of intuition. Number three in my cons column was the impact of a positive result on Murph. I was concerned that he would feel guilty, however irrationally, as I would have done if I'd been him. This toxic inheritance wasn't like passing on eye colour.

My friends were also divided into pro and con camps. Some were temperamentally opposed to false consciousness and the idea of 'living a lie'. Others were convinced that this knowledge, which could never be un-known, would make the years before I developed symptoms unbearable. Would finding out what lay in store for me ruin my present? Ambivalent and indecisive, I flip-flopped a hundred times a day, wishing once again that Susan could have been there to talk things through with me. I'm sure she would have supported me whatever I decided, but she would also have made it very clear whether she was pro or con. I think she would have been pro, as she was always good at confronting hard truths. In a different mood, I was glad she'd died before this era of hard-to-bear revelations. Murph hadn't told her about his mother or his at-risk status, so she'd gone to her grave blissfully unaware of the genequake that was about to shake the foundations of our family.

I read everything I could find about HD; this caused many sleepless nights, but it was important to be fully apprised of the facts so I could make an informed decision about whether to take the test. I read everything online and in print, including memoirs by people caring for relatives with HD and a biography of folk legend Woody Guthrie, whose mother had HD and passed it on to him. She sounded scary, aggressive and compulsive, with no parenting skills. I felt sorry for Woody when I read that she had set fire to his childhood home, but comforted myself with the thought that his compassion and fellow feeling may have been nurtured in the same house. I would have been proud to share my malformed Huntingtin protein with him – as opposed to, say, Frank Sinatra.

All this reading confirmed my worst fears. What a terrible burden I would be ... and who was going to look after me? Tom wouldn't be able to give up work and I wouldn't want him to. But how would we be able to afford a carer when I got to the point of needing one? We'd need to sell the house. And what about my daughter?

Once I knew all this I wanted to un-know it, but it took up residence in my consciousness and proved difficult to shift. Needless to say, Dan had not been googling HD or seeking out online forums where at-risk people unburdened themselves and commiserated with each other; characteristically, he'd imposed an information blackout on himself from the moment I told him about about Murph's diagnosis. Was he more or less anxious than me? He certainly spent less time in tears. But I did all that research because I wanted to find evidence that my depressive nature was making me doom myself unnecessarily. How would my optimistic husband have reacted if he'd been in my position? Tom would have found a way to enjoy life while he still could and focused on the here and now, planting some hardy perennials in the back garden and teaching our daughter to sail.

I lacked the inner resources for HD. Being me rather than Tom, I was lost in brooding negativity and blamed myself for my inability to escape my automatic thoughts. I projected myself into a future where I acted like the people I'd read about on the forums, propositioning my husband in front of my children and scaring their school friends.

I found a list of pros and cons for taking the test on the Huntington's Disease Association website. Pros: increased ability to plan for the future and make informed reproductive choices; relief of uncertainty and worry. Cons: fear of mutation-positive result; lack of a cure; worry about genetic discrimination; preference for living in hope.

I hadn't thought about the possibility of genetic discrimination – in fact, I had to google it to find out what it even was. It happens when people are treated differently by an employer or insurance company because they have a gene mutation that causes or increases the risk of an inherited disorder. Without an employer or insurance, that was one con I could cross off the list. We did talk a lot about our reproductive options, though, and our feelings, which I found harder to talk about than Tom.

In February 2007, when Anna was three, I finally made up my mind and went to Queen Mary's Hospital near Paddington to have the test, knowing I could pull out at any point if I wanted to. After all the delay and deliberation, there was something incongruous about how quick and hitch-free the process of actually getting tested was. I almost found myself feeling a little foolish for having made such a fuss about it.

To distract ourselves while we waited for the results, we booked into a family-friendly hotel in the Bedruthan Steps area of Cornwall for a minibreak. It was a long way from London – should we drive or get the train? Tom thought the train would be less arduous as Anna was often sick in cars. The journey there was lengthy but without incident, and we arrived in good order. The hotel was reassuringly normal-looking (I had worried that there would be too many wipe-clean surfaces) and our bedroom big and pleasant with a good sea view. Tom suggested a walk on the beach because he thinks fresh air is a universal panacea, and for once I wasn't going to argue with him. Anna toddled cutely down the path after us, a picture of innocence from a Palmolive ad. The next day I felt strong enough to brave the soft play area, then regretted it. I left Tom there with Anna and went to find somewhere to smoke.

Dinners were comically disrupted by the sounds of other people's children crying. There was a baby monitor on almost every table. Anna wouldn't settle so we went backwards and forwards to our room. All the other couples were enjoying themselves, unfazed. There was a crèche so we left Anna there for a couple of hours while we went to the hotel spa. No one else was there. I have never felt closer to Tom. Whatever happened, we were in this together. I wished I could have sweated out my anxiety in the sauna, though.

The night before we were due to leave, I didn't sleep at all. Our appointment with the HD specialist nurse was at 5 p.m. the next day. We had carefully planned our journey home, to minimise stress and build in some contingency time (Murph always recommended this), but the fates were conspiring against us from the off. The taxi was late picking us up so the driver had to really floor it to get us to the station in time. Anna was sick in the back as we hurtled around the twisty country lanes. I was in tears the whole way and furious with the driver, who charged extra for cleaning up the sick. Then the train broke down just outside Plymouth and had to be shunted back to the station. By now I was near-hysterical as we were taken off the stricken train and left on the windswept platform.

Plymouth was where Murph had been brought up, so being held there against our will when we were trying to move forward had a horrible resonance; I felt like I'd stumbled into an implausibly scripted melodrama. Eventually we were herded onto another train, but it was already full so we had to stand for hours.

We got a taxi from Paddington to the hospital. My best friend was waiting in reception to look after Anna while we went to see the nurse. I was in tears as we sat down and explained the drama of our journey there. I couldn't read the nurse's expression. Then she said, 'Well, I'm sorry to have to make a bad day worse ... '

I did have the HD gene. What was there to do but cry? Normally stoical Tom looked stricken. There were tissues on the table but they weren't thick enough for my man-sized outpourings. They brought us sweet, milky tea but I could only manage a couple of sips. I hate tea with milk in. Was this what the future would taste like? Did it mark the start of an era of sickly consolations that were kindly meant but ill judged? The nurse was checking discreetly whether I was suicidal before letting us go. Did we have enough support? Possibly not. I was no longer in therapy.

Lottie – who had recently become my stepmother, so was now literally also called Charlotte Raven – flew unbidden into my mind in the likeness of a black crow with green fingers (she blogged as 'The Galloping Gardener'), but no matter, I shooed her away … I wasn't ready for her to know. At least Tom and I had each other, for the moment, though I knew the result would test our relationship. There were already hairline fractures in it that weren't visible to anyone but us.

My friend gathered us up. We were all crying in the taxi back to ours, which upset Anna.

People tried to be reassuring. Tom's mum said, 'Look on the bright side – you might not get it for ages,' because Murph hadn't had any symptoms until he was in his sixties. What she didn't realise was that his was a very unusual case. It's much more common for HD to arrive in your late thirties or early forties, when you are just getting settled. His getting it late did not in any way imply that I would too – in fact, the number of repetitions of the faulty gene made it more likely that I would get it earlier.

When I called Murph to tell him, I was surprised to find him weirdly detached and unempathic. He just said, 'Don't worry about it. It takes ages to develop.' I understood that he was trying to be kind but he wasn't reflecting my reality. The degenerative process can be so slow in late-onset HD that it is often mistaken for signs of ageing. The younger you are, the faster it burns through you.

The way I saw it, the cognitive impairments alone would derail my life. More than anything else I was scared of not being able to think – I wouldn't mind shaking or stumbling if I could still land a punch intellectually. The books in my study embodied my identity. I was also worried about being a terrible mother to Anna. We had planned to have another child, but this now seemed irresponsible given that they would have a 50 per cent chance of inheriting the gene mutation.

I never regretted getting tested – it was a calculated gamble, rationally founded. But I did wonder afterwards if my approach to making the decision had been the right one. Perhaps I should have trusted my intuition more than my pros and cons list. If I had used my gut to guide me, would the outcome have been the same? Probably. I sense that my impulse to bring things into the light would have shepherded me along the same path, towards the truth. Susan would have been proud.

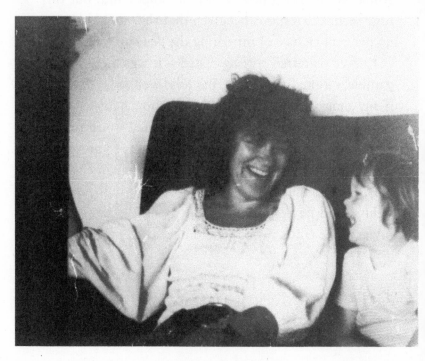

Susan and me, aged four

Forward to socialism!
KEVIN

Name _Charlotte Rauon_
Subject _Rough_
Form _U4G_

PHILIP & TACEY LTD England

ambrella

UNITY IS STRENGTH

Girls' Public Day School Trust

Brighton scooter girls 1984

BRIGHTON & HOVE HIGH SCHOOL

Vespa

ROUGH BOOK

Victory to the miners!

THE WORKERS UNITED WILL NEVER BE DEFEATED!

My militant era exercise book

2

Normalcy

Before HD crashed into my life I was lucky enough to have a job I loved that allowed me to express myself, yet still brought in enough money to waste on clothes. My career in journalism was a seat-of-the-pants perform-ance, though, and I was constantly worried about being exposed as a fraud.

I'd left journalism school in a huff halfway through the course, without ever having got the hang of short-hand. The Westminster Press MA was inauspiciously located in the basement of a dingy office block on the seafront at Hastings. We learned how to write news using acrostics, and there were lessons on dark jour-nalistic arts like doorstepping. But I resented the way they kept telling me I would need to 'do my time' as a reporter on a local paper before I could expect to get anywhere, and as for the dress code ... We were told to look professional, so trooped down the hill to 'the office' in skirt suits and sensible shoes every morning. This wasn't how I'd imagined my life when my teen-age self had cast me as one of the sophisticated beau monde.

I left because I felt that there must be a way into journalism that didn't involve quite so many trips to M&S, although this may just have been a cover for the fact that I was finding it tough going. After a few months of moping around my old childhood bedroom in Brighton, I thought about my options. I felt I had something to say but my thinking was woolly after a long spell at the academic coalface, deconstructing everything that came into view – the habits I'd picked up on the Critical Theory MA course I completed before going to journalism school were proving hard to shake. My writing was elliptical with Derridean flourishes, which I was quite proud of. I'd never actually read Derrida or Lacan, relying instead on the Fontana Modern Masters series of books I'd had to hand when writing essays but never brought to class. It had seemed to work, and my tutors never guessed that I was cribbing – even when I borrowed whole phrases from the Modern Masters without attribution.

But this approach would only work for an academic audience. I wanted to be *read*! I'd long been a fan of Julie Burchill's writing, and aspired to her level of clarity. She was also the editor-in-chief of my favourite magazine, the *Modern Review*. Everyone was still talking about postmodernism in the early 90s, and my time with the Modern Masters had left me well equipped for these conversations. I wrote a heavily ironic letter to Toby Young, the editor of the *Modern Review*, which took me ages to compose. I was delighted when he called to offer me work experience, just in time to rescue me from my provincial fate. The bright lights of London beckoned. I was nervous, though – the *Modern Review* could be intimidatingly clever, so I pictured its office as a kind of modern-day Algonquin where wit was weaponised.

Toby Young ran the magazine from the front room of his house in Shepherd's Bush. Its 'low culture for high-brows' credo was timely, but at that point we didn't realise we were the trailblazers for a large-scale cultural shift. The section editors were Oxbridge graduates and mostly men. There was no scanner, so all the articles had to be transcribed – by me. I didn't do very much work, which annoyed the deputy editor who ended up picking up the slack. He didn't stay up all night, so he was always in earlier than me, clucking disapprovingly. They printed my hard-to-decipher articles with minimal editing. Even I couldn't understand my book reviews, the piece about that boyband I was into or my paean to a new cultural form, reality TV.

But I got noticed by the right people, and was soon delighted to find myself descending the Titanic-like staircase of the Atlantic Bar and Grill in Piccadilly with Julie Burchill. My memory is hazy. Beautiful people in sharp suits and bodycon dresses were downing sea breezes, smoking and delivering killer lines simultan-eously, which I suppose is what passes for multitasking in a decadent boom time. If you can remember the 90s, you weren't really there; I remember so little of it that I must have been more there than practically anyone, Liam Gallagher excepted. It was a hedonistic era, and I was fully committed to being zeitgeisty.

Julie and I ended up in a relationship. Our first date was to a press screening of the film *Heavenly Creatures*, which was apt. We giggled all the way through, infuriating all the critics who were actually trying to review it. My main memory of living together is arguing incessantly about the death penalty. I chucked her out but then she married my brother, so I've never completely got rid of her.

The 90s was also a golden age for journalism, because the money was still good and they gave you plenty of time to think. I managed to stay quite highbrow for a while, writing about the intersection of politics and popular culture as I had for the *Modern Review*. In spite of my good intentions, though, I soon found myself accepting a commission from *Cosmopolitan* to write a piece in praise of stupid men. Wracked with remorse about dumbing myself down, I sought out the *Guardian*'s women's editor and wrote a couple of pieces for her about 'fauxminimism' and girl power. She was pleased with my counterintuitive broadsides and I was promoted.

As a columnist in the New Labour era, I should have been able to find plenty of interesting things to write about, but I actually seemed to run out of subjects alarmingly quickly. I was redeployed as a controversialist, paid to criticise and take issue. When they moved my column from the women's page to G2 it was a bit better paid but a lot less edifying. I had become a knee-jerk iconoclast, set on attack mode with the complacent bourgeoisie in my sights, including but not limited to *Guardian* readers.

The persona I had arrived at was perpetually angry, arguing for argument's sake, never pausing for thought, heedless of the impact my critiques might have on the people I took down. I condemned the whole city of Liverpool for mourning one of their own, saying they were sentimentalists who revelled in their victimhood (I had planned to write a less incendiary version of the same piece but a *Times* columnist had beaten me to it, so I'd felt obliged to amplify the point). I got into terrible trouble for that, but why had they published it in the first place? They wanted their commentators to sail close to the wind, then abandoned them when they did. When people complained to the editor, the paper didn't support me; in a pre-social media era, I was hung out to dry on the letters page. I tried to be unrepentant but was secretly mortified.

A few weeks later I was nearly sacked for plagiarism. My piece about The Beatles had indeed borrowed a few phrases from something I may have glanced at in the *NME*, but I maintained that I'd had the idea of slagging them off first.

Even my cultural commentary was confrontational. My book reviews were polemics; I always knew what I wanted to say about the author so would simply speed-read for evidence of my theory, never taking anything in. Interviews were the same. I interviewed Bret Easton Ellis in a minimalist hotel – he was one of my literary heroes but when I listened to the tape it was only me talking, inviting him to agree with my idea of his most famous work.

Susan was my biggest fan. She cut out all my pieces and pasted them into scrapbooks. She was angry with my critics, as she had been with my teachers when I'd behaved badly at school – defending the indefensible. I had gone to a private secondary school in Brighton with a bottle-green uniform that I adapted when I was in my mod phase, then my goth phase. Every few weeks Susan would be called into the headmistress's office for a dressing-down. Some of the parents were concerned that I wasn't giving their daughters 'room to grow'. I wasn't exactly a bully, just overbearing and arguing with everyone about everything. If I'd been in a state school my oppositional position wouldn't have made any sense, and I would have come across bigger personalities than mine. It suited me to stay in a school where I believed making my form teacher cry and not doing any actual work ever were radical acts.

Susan blamed the school for oppressing me because of my political views; they were trying to crush my subversive spirit. It was a point of principle to her that I should never be told off. The miners' strike of 1984 helped turn a passing interest in politics into something more like a fixation. To demonstrate their broadmindedness, the school invited two of the miners who'd been staying with us during the strike (they were picketing a local power station) to debate with one of the fathers, who was a manager at the National Coal Board. I cried when the strike ended.

Before school each morning, Susan would backcomb my blonde hair into a beehive. When I shifted my subcultural affiliation she helped me dye my hair black and crimped it for me – a labour of love, like all our collaborations. I was a perfectionist about my look, so it took ages to get it right and I was often late for school. For Susan, child-centred parenting meant always deferring to me; lacking confidence herself, she would never have imagined you could have too much of the wrong kind. I ruled the roost, believing I was more qualified for that position than any of the adults in the house, and developed an iron will that could not be contradicted.

On one holiday to the US when I was about fourteen, Murph organised a cheering crowd to meet me at the airport, waving signs bearing my name. We drove to his friend's factory and I gave an impromptu speech to all the workers there, which they duly applauded. I still have a plaque that reads: 'Charlotte Raven – in gratitude from the American people.' My parents thought this was the best way to treat me and I loved it.

I thought Murph was a capitalist pig, like Mr Clean in The Jam's song. He was the managing director of a group of trade publications, foremost of which was the venerable *International Tax-Free Trader*. Duty-free was small beer in the 80s, but large enough to have conferences in nice places (and at least he didn't work on *Tableware International* – the freebies would have been wedding-list china). Unmaterialistic Susan was unexcited by the bribes for wives that tended to be handed out at such events, so I amassed a fine collection of high-end knick-knacks on my dressing table. I never saw any contradiction between my Marxism and my love of expensive perfume.

But we disrespected Murph, in the very house where he paid all the bills. Compared with the revolutionary and/or creative life, his job seemed like a silly way to make a living. When he got home from work we were usually watching *Coronation Street*, so he'd be greeted with an emphatic 'Shush'. But somehow this never seemed to bother him; he was a benign facilitator, always refilling everyone's glasses. My mother and I were members of the Militant tendency, an entryist Trotskyite organisation attached parasitically to the Labour Party (Susan eventually fell out with them for calling a school students' strike that I participated in. My headmistress came to get me from the rally!). Murph was kind and respectful to every extremist who crossed the threshold, making them all feel welcome. A friend from that era said he was 'the most likeable capitalist you could ever hope to meet'.

I sensed Susan's frustration about being an executive wife. She read voraciously, as if her life depended on it. As soon as we left home, she went straight back into education. She'd originally left school at fifteen, but she eventually got a PhD in Masculinities. She actively discouraged Murph from inviting work colleagues round for dinner, and her housework was not of the highest standard. She hated going to duty-free symposiums, where she would inevitably be patronised by unreconstructed men. On one memorable occasion, she got into a heated argument with the CEO of a cigarette company about mutually assured destruction. A couple of witnesses have told me that her reasoned and informed case for unilateral nuclear disarmament won the day; Marlboro Man conceded defeat.

Because of Susan, I grew up convinced that learning how to boil an egg would lead to a life of domestic servitude. We lived on Findus crispy pancakes and fish fingers; she kept me out of the kitchen and cleared up around me. The dream we shared was that I would be a childless writer when I grew up. We visited the Brontës' house in Haworth every couple of years, walking to Top Withens, where *Wuthering Heights* was set. I was named after Charlotte Brontë.

In the last few months of her life, Susan was worried about me. I was struggling with the book of doom and my relationship with her had entered a new phase that we were both finding it hard to adjust to. After years of calling her twice a day to keep her in the loop about my life, I had become semi-detached. Being in therapy had given me a new perspective on my upbringing. A slight change in the light had allowed me to see that we were unhealthily enmeshed. Ruling the roost had been as bad for me as it had for everyone else. I didn't blame Susan, but my tactical withdrawal was understandably painful for her. She died after a failed heart bypass operation on Valentine's Day 2001, so we never had a chance to sort it all out.

A couple of months later I moved to a house in Kentish Town that was slightly too big for me. To keep me company I bought a puppy, then panicked when it turned out to be even needier than I was. I wasn't ready for the responsibility (you can't leave them alone when you go to the pub!), so felt pleased for both of us when I found a loving family to take him off my hands. But I still wanted some sort of pet with dog-like attributes to share my life. Susan had always been a cat person and a fan of Maine Coons in particular. She had two with puritan names who used to sit like sentinels on the arms of her chair, breathing in her cigarette smoke. But Prudence and Constance would be staying in Brighton, so I contacted a Maine Coon breeder on the south coast.

Once there, I had to restrain myself for fear I might become the mad cat lady of Kentish Town: there were adorable kittens in baskets, on the floor, on every surface. I would have taken as many as I could fit in the car, had they not been so prohibitively priced. In the end I came back with two sisters. I wanted to call them Grace and Abounding after John Bunyan's puritan treatise, then lost my nerve.

A mutual friend introduced me to Tom at a party in Notting Hill in 2002. All the men in my life up to that point had been dysfunctional to varying degrees, but it was clear from the outset that Tom was both sane and interesting. Our first night together was a drunken laugh. There were no dating apps in those days – we just busked romance. It was hit and miss but more enjoyable for it. What would Tom have put on his profile? Would I have found his passion for Fulham Football Club off-putting? There was also the question of his taste in clothes: I was a style fascist with an image to maintain, and wouldn't normally have been seen dead on a date with someone in Berghaus trousers.

But when he was speaking, all the other people in the room faded to grey. It really was love at first chat, and after a couple of lines of coke I started to feel as though we could literally conquer the world together. I had never experienced such an intense connection with anyone before. He even made football seem fascinating! I was pleased to see my narrow-mindedness and self-limiting beliefs disappear between the sofa cushions. We had so much in common. His favourite song was 'Another Girl, Another Planet' by The Only Ones – that's *my* favourite song! At that point, the little areas of difference still seemed interesting rather than threatening.

We kissed on top of the coats in the spare room. When we got back to my house, one of the kittens had shat on the spare bed. In the morning I wanted a McDonald's breakfast. We both had hangovers, but Tom set off up the high street in search of Egg McMuffins. He got lost on the way back. I was worried he wouldn't return, and there were a few anxious minutes of actually missing him. This little scene introduced all the major themes of our subsequent relationship. Tom was brought up to be dutiful, even if it meant subordinating his own wishes, and I was raised to be bossy and needy. This dynamic was played out from the early hours of our relationship to its conclusion many years later. Looking back on it now, I wish I'd got dressed instead of lying there like the Queen of Sheba. We could have gone to McDonald's together. What could have begun as a collaborative partnership was skewed in my favour from the start.

Our second non-date was at a seafood restaurant in Brixton. There were live lobsters in tanks, and Tom entertained me with tales from the field (he made anthropological documentaries). In his twenties he had lived in the Burmese jungle with a minority who were fighting for independence from the military dictatorship. He had a well-thought-through radical critique of anthropology, and a radical critique of the radical critique. It was great to feel my horizons broaden after years of limiting parochialism. Just as importantly, we were politically aligned. There was just one important area of concern: he was wearing leather trousers. With a white shirt tucked in. Needless to say, the effect wasn't Jaggeresque. I was mightily relieved to discover that he at least had a motorbike parked outside.

The day after, I ran into a friend at the Festival Hall and told him I'd met the person I was going to marry. I'd never thought about marrying anyone before. Scrolling back through all my relationships, I could see that none of my exes would have made good fathers, even if they'd been the marrying kind. Once I'd decided this, I thought it would only be a matter of time before Tom was persuaded, by force of argument, that I was the right woman for him. Soon after that, he went away to Ethiopia to film a documentary but, encouragingly, sent me love letters and poems. We talked for hours whenever he was in range, running up a huge bill at his end.

In due course he moved from his flat in Brixton to my house in Kentish Town. I felt so safe with him, even on the back of his motorbike (much safer than when I was driving my own car). We cruised around London in what felt like an endless summer. Unexpectedly, life had become open-topped. Tom's optimism was infectious. I started to feel that it might be possible to redeem myself, that the next chapter of my life could be fun, ethically sourced and directed by a robust moral compass.

A year later, Tom and I were in Skye on a minibreak with a friend and her soon-to-be-ex-husband (they split up while we were there). We'd spent the whole weekend arguing. I was impatient for romantic avowals, or a full explanation of why he hadn't proposed to me yet. Surely he knew everything about me by then?

I had form when it came to demanding presents before they could be freely given. Murph always gave me money for my birthday, which is in September. The amount increased as he got richer, rising to but possibly not peaking at £1,000. Instead of waiting, I would call him in August and ask him to transfer it. Or July. In Skye, I wanted Tom to advance his marriage proposal in exactly the same way. But my nagging had the opposite effect, and we nearly split up – no one likes to be chivvied, especially about getting married. Things were looking dicey on the way home but then, in the baggage reclaim area and probably still feeling ambivalent about me, he produced a diamond that he'd had on him the whole time. When we got in the car, we both felt cheated of the moment he had planned as a memory to cherish. But it was all my fault.

I often wonder whether this kind of unreasonable and ultimately self-defeating behaviour was a product of my upbringing, HD or a combination of the two. From my point of view it would be far easier to blame

HD than myself or Susan and Murph, but I can't help thinking that I wasn't symptomatic when I was being horrible to Tom; I may have been prematurely unempathic as a result of the disease, but that's no excuse for throwing your weight around. And it can't really have been HD that made me a stroppier-than-average teenager, because it would be extremely unusual for anyone to become symptomatic at such a young age. I just wasn't a very nice person.

Meeting Tom had been transformative. Susan's dream of me being a childless writer had been replaced by my own vision of the future, where it was possible to have both children and a creative life. My thinking had changed; rather than distracting me, the presence of children might be enriching. I could picture them sitting around our kitchen table, joining the conversation. They might even be fun at parties.

I married Tom in 2003, at the Old Ship Hotel in Brighton. It was the finale of a long-running production of 90s excess, a last hurrah before I settled down. My feminist friends were worried when I revealed my wedding plans to them. I thought I was aiming for an edgy and modern take on a wedding rather than a puffed-sleeved fairy tale like Princess Diana's, but for some reason it ended up more traditional than billed. From the moment I booked the wedding planners to the last song of the party at my family home, the script was a bride-focused fantasy in which Tom was marginalised. We did agree that Brighton would be the best setting for the wedding and we both liked the Old Ship Hotel, because although it was run-down it had charm and character; the faded function room upstairs looked like a blank canvas and I felt confident that it could be moulded into the grand design I had in mind. I didn't care if the food was horrible, as that was much less important than the setting.

That was the last decision we made together. I didn't want his large extended family there so I didn't invite them. Murph paid for everything and the bills began to mount up several months before my big day. There were Eve Lom facials to make my skin radiant. My hair was designed by my Bond Street hairdresser, a long time in advance. My Vera Wang wedding dress came from Liberty. Susan's best friend, who'd come with me to choose it, cried when she saw me in it, so that was 'the one'. It had a train and a veil, which I was going to decide about on the day. For good measure and enhanced bling, I bought a crystal tiara which sparkled like diamonds in the bridal shop – but my hair design had to be revised in light of this, which meant more appointments and more expense for Murph. I couldn't decide between two pairs of Louboutin shoes in the shop so I bought both and kept one in reserve.

The planners helped me with a colour scheme for the bridesmaids' dresses, and my dressmaker made them without consulting any of the people who were going to be shoehorned into them. The lilac monstrosities were fine for the three-year-old but not for my grown-up friend, who hated hers. I still made her wear it.

As the big day approached, I became Bridezilla; I was furious with the wedding planners for ordering the wrong type of ivory for the tablecloths but had to let it go. For our wedding night I booked a room with no view in Brighton's first boutique hotel, which was going to be more expensive than staying at The Old Ship but also, clearly, much hipper. Everything was falling into place. Making the table plan was fun as the guests were an interesting melange of media people and friends from the high-end therapy groups I'd been attending (only the good-looking ones, though). I was pleased by the calibre of my various signings, which included the CEO of Issey Miyake.

Waking up on my wedding day in my childhood bedroom, my first thoughts were of Tom and what the tuxedos he had hired from Austin Reed at the last minute were going to look like; I had to speak sternly with myself until I remembered what I was meant to be doing that day and how pleased I was to be marrying him, whatever the tuxedos looked like. I really loved him and was looking forward to our future as a team of two. I still missed Susan, though, so my emotions were bitter-sweet for the first few hours. She would have approved of Tom but not the crystal tiara. As a concession to her I decided not to wear the veil, which was the right decision. Murph said, 'Why would you want to cover your face? You look beautiful.' He never normally said anything like that.

We had a woman celebrant and I was pleased with the vows in the end. The readings were as far from cliché as it was possible to be. An old friend I met on my critical theory MA read a passage from Heidegger that went down very well.

The food wasn't very nice but no one cared. Tom spoke, my reluctant bridesmaid spoke and Tom's best man spoke. Why didn't I? I had prepared something to say but felt too emotional to deliver it. I was enraptured.

Poor Murph – after making him pay for everything and walk me down the aisle, I even made him change his speech. He'd been planning something corporate and bland that didn't mention Susan and quoted extensively from the beloved *Speaker's Treasury of Quotations* he always consulted before making speeches at duty-free symposia. We went to the beach to have our pictures taken and he looked unsteady on his feet, as if a strong wind could have carried him away.

In the early days of my marriage to Tom I was hypercritical about everything and everyone, including his friends and family. Being paid to be horrible about people caused a lot of collateral damage to my relationships. It would be no exaggeration to say that I nearly argued myself out of a marriage.

My opposition to him having a social life was argued on a case-by-case basis. The friend who'd introduced us had become a bit of a boaster, so wasn't allowed across the threshold. Someone he'd met at university who'd become an internet entrepreneur had been cast out on political grounds. Another friend wanted us to play parlour games at her thirtieth birthday, so I made Tom drive me home (I hate parlour games). Tom's family liked playing Consequences on Christmas Day, which I scorned (there were no Christmas traditions in my family, apart from drinking too much and watching TV). So I'd sit it out, tutting.

I didn't want him to enjoy himself unless he was with me or in my milieu. When he did manage to prise himself away for an evening, I would text him compulsively. It was airless and oppressive. If we went out with his friends, I would dress to kill everyone in range. My favoured outfits were all aggressive statements of sartorial disdain, like the sculptural 'pieces' by Issey Miyake which made me resemble a negative of the Pierrot from David Bowie's 'Ashes to Ashes' video (they didn't take up much room in my wardrobe, so I saw no reason not to just keep on buying them). Tom preferred the 'flirty and feminine' Betsey Johnson dress I'd bought but never worn.

We had plenty of space but I wanted to upsize. I found what looked like my idea of a forever home on a lovely corner plot in a street with cherry blossom on the trees. At first sight it looked more like a party house than a family home. The owner, a chain-smoking architect with an interest in crop circles, had brought up his family there. When he invited us round for drinks to assess our suitability (we were up against a couple of other families), I felt quietly confident that Tom would charm him into a deal. It worked, and we got the house.

While we were renovating it, I found out I was pregnant. I went to a few pregnancy yoga classes in Primrose Hill but had to stop because it felt too much like a middle-class cliché.

We nearly came to blows about the price of the wallpaper I had sourced, from a company whose designs hang in the Pugin Room at the Palace of Westminster. The grand, gilt-edged mirror the architect had left us looked equally amazing. I pictured our hallway as the entrance to a Victorian opium den. The white carpets on the stairs and landings weren't child friendly.

We had some great parties there, despite the fact that mine and Tom's entrance policies could hardly have been more different. Mine was selective: I wanted the guests to reflect my image of myself at that time. Tom was a more generous host, with a more inclusive vision that did not involve dress codes or elaborate background checks. He was interested in people, and had a talent for making everyone feel like honoured guests whose presence was crucial to creating party alchemy. He was most himself at parties, because he was a social animal who came from a big family. When he was growing up, his parents had often rolled back the carpets in the living room to jive on the parquet.

Everyone loved Tom's anecdotes about his misspent youth listening to Led Zeppelin on acid, and I was pleased to be creating material for the stories he would tell in the future.

One party will give you a flavour of them all, as they have merged in my memory. At his insistence, Tom's old friend's bearded hippy partner was there. And that strange old university friend of mine Tom had inherited when I stopped answering his calls. A journalist friend was saying I was mad to consider giving up my column to write a book; a newspaper executive was ejected for lunging at one of my friends. After everyone had gone, me and Tom stayed up talking until dawn. There was always so much to say. And in the morning, amazingly, he never minded clearing up, no matter how hungover he was.

Feeling professionally invincible, I decided to press ahead with my book idea – that feminist conduct book for girls, which was commissioned in short order. I thought it would take me six months to write, and spent my advance in two hours on Bond Street. A few weeks later, when I saw some covetable colour-block pieces in the Jil Sander sale on South Molton Street, I had to ask Tom to lend me the money to buy them.

I was terrible with money, especially other people's. I'd never learned how to budget. Whenever I got into debt, whether by a few hundred or a few thousand, Murph would always bail me out. At university he'd paid off my overdraft whenever I spent too much on partying and clothes, and this carried on seamlessly into adulthood. When he came up to visit us from Brighton, I used to take him to Liberty with me. He'd sit on a velvet chair in Women's Wear while I tried on a selection of edgy designer pieces. And it wasn't just clothes – he also paid for the York flagstones in our refurbished back garden and the new coal-look fire in the sitting room. In spite of his largesse, though, he wasn't comfortable talking about money. Susan must have found it difficult too. They never had a joint account so she was given 'housekeeping money' every week in cash, and he never told her anything about the bigger financial picture.

Tom paid for the independent midwives who attended Anna's home birth in 2005, two years after we got married. The NHS midwives I'd come across were either saints or sadists, and I couldn't risk the latter being on shift when

I went into labour. Committing to a home birth meant giving birth without any pain relief apart from gas and air; everyone who knew me thought this was mad and uncharacteristic. Many of them tried to talk me out of it. It wasn't as if I was opposed to drugs – why would I want a natural birth when I took drugs for every low-level complaint, and even just to cheer myself up? I knew they were wrong, right up to the moment when I had my first contraction. By that time it was too late to go to hospital.

Fourteen hours later I was still in the sitting room, cursing my teacher at the active birth centre who had said that pain was a matter of perception. I gave birth in a pool and the midwife took a picture. When it was all over, I wanted a McDonald's. The midwife (rather than Tom) went to get me a Big Mac, which has never tasted better before or since. They wouldn't have done that in a hospital.

Tom's parents were our first visitors. After what I'd just been through, I was expecting to be the focus of attention rather than the baby. But the gifts were all for Anna. It took a couple of months to adjust to having someone in the house whose needs took priority over mine. I'd read a lot of books while I was pregnant, but only one of them still felt relevant. Not the book on attachment parenting but the one by Rachel Cusk that portrayed motherhood as a moment of self-erasure, not fulfilment. Everyone had been outraged when it first came out, feeling sorry for the never-named baby, but I'd identified with the writer. It took a while for my narcissistic wound to heal. Anna came slowly into view. Then I fell in love with her.

3

Lost

There's an art to losing and being lost that I have never mastered. When I lose things, I always look in the places they're least likely to be first. If my mobile phone isn't in the basket with the cat food, the box file in my study or my knicker drawer, it *might* be on the sideboard, where it's meant to be. Hope is still alive at this point; I might still find it. If I tried the sideboard first I would see that it wasn't there and panic. Then there would be no point looking in out-of-the-way places, so I might as well spend the rest of the morning in tears on the phone to the mobile company, asking for a replacement.

This strategy protects me from the trauma of loss, but it also wastes a lot of time. I never have time to write because I'm always looking for things in weird places, getting more and more agitated. I can't relax until I've found them and I often don't. I'm always mourning something.

Someone once described HD as an illness of mourning, which seems very apt. You lose your identity, and some of your humanity, while remaining aware enough to keep a tally of every loss. To be thrown off the familiar path with no map takes a stout heart and an ability to get interested in the diversions. If I was more like Tom I might have seen losing the components of my front-facing persona and ability to engage in intellectual projects as an opportunity, but I don't think even he would have been able to put a positive spin on the loss of his bearings.

For me, it started with small, unexplained absences: my car keys, my glasses, a million lighters, shoes, clothes. Then I lost the world, city by city. Familiar places I'd felt confident navigating became a scary tangle of streets, so I stayed in the house. Then the car itself started to go missing: when we stopped at services I could never find my way back to it. Bigger human losses followed. I lost my sexuality. Friends stopped remembering to visit me. And then I began to lose my own past: as my short- and long-term memory were affected by HD, the story of my life receded into the distance and became increasingly inaccessible to me.

Before all those losses, I was living as fully as one could with the prospect of total identity collapse looming over one. We tried to stay positive and focus on building our family in the form we'd intended. There was one gain: our son John, who was born on a lovely day in April. It took us a long time to decide whether and how to have another child, now that we knew they would have a 50 per cent chance of inheriting the gene mutation. There were many things to consider. I didn't want Anna to be an only child, coping with weird me and having no one to play with. Among the heartbreaking accounts I'd read from the children of HD parents was one from a girl called Lily, who'd said that growing up with her mother had been like living with a ghost – she was there but never emotionally present. Lost and present at the same time, which must have been difficult for everyone. Lily couldn't work out why her home wasn't full of love and laughter like those of her friends; she didn't find out what was wrong with her mother until much later.

Instead of breaking out the pros and cons list, we examined our consciences. Could we justify bringing another child into the world, knowing what was in store for them? It might have been desirable, but was it right to carry on conceiving regardless? I wasn't very maternal in any case and would soon be much less so. In the end, instinct won over argument and I found myself in the unexpected position of longing for another baby as other women seem to but I never had. There might even have been a hope for redemption in the mix of emotions, a sense that 'choosing life' might have a good karmic payoff. We briefly considered IVF – advances in gene science mean it's possible to select an embryo without the HD gene – but it would have been a long and fraught process. We decided, perhaps irresponsibly, that trying to procreate the old-fashioned way would be more fun.

Tom's job in TV meant he was often away for long stretches. He wasn't rooted to one chair as I was, or even one continent. And he always seemed to work in places where there was no mobile phone signal. My cousin wondered aloud whether Tom's failure to pick up my texts or return my calls might mean he didn't want to. Go figure, he said. It did seem odd, I thought – the whole world was connected and Wi-Fi was everywhere but, for whatever reason, Tom would disappear off the radar for weeks on end. If he wasn't working on a pared-to-the-bone reality TV programme on a desert island in Panama he'd be filming a rain-lashed trawler crew in the middle of the North Sea, or trekking to an abandoned Soviet research station in an area of Antarctica that is literally called The Pole of Inaccessibility. Go figure!

Was he trying to give me the slip? I wouldn't have blamed him, as it can't have been much fun having me soldered to his side. Tom likes getting lost at festivals. He is a utopian for whom festivals are a microcosm of an ideal society, where people show their best selves – a post-capitalist fantasy where difference is celebrated and every conversation and random encounter is alive with possibility. We used to go to the same festival at Port Eliot with the family every year, but every year it got a bit more stressful. Whatever the weather, the same thing always happened: I'd lose my phone, my bag, my money, my tent (quite a feat in daylight) and then myself, multiple times. I could never understand the map or the festival programme, or even ask people for directions. I had no sense of time passing. I'd get so confused about the filigree of intersecting arrangements – and the more confused I got, the more anxious I felt.

The last time we went, Tom was conflicted about all the middle-class festival goers forming orderly queues for Monmouth Coffee. In the old days, festivals had been ramshackle affairs with no big headline acts or sanitiser, perfect for improvisers and wanderers like him. He remembers when the doors of perception at Stonehenge and Glastonbury were mere catflaps, and the atmosphere of post-punk menace on the traveller scene at festivals in the late 80s. Through it all, Tom was probably just sitting in someone's tent, talking shit in the same clothes he'd arrived in. He thought of disorientation as a state of mind replete with possibility, not an uncomfortable side effect.

The modern, family-friendly festival is fun but we all have each other's coordinates. This is progress, from my point of view, but I can see that it's a completely different proposition. You can't really lose yourself; I still get paranoid and anxious, but most people don't. You will be tracked or texted. There is a place for lost children. Places to charge your phone. People get elegantly wasted rather than trashed, and no one ever smudges their mascara.

I only noticed one gurning drug casualty the last time we were there, and people were sneering at him. Being out of your head in an unattractive way was clearly *de trop*. He was even wearing a shell suit – *imagine!* This ghost of festivals past was delivering a message, but it wasn't getting through to the middle-aged fashionistas or their manicured progeny. Only Tom was listening.

Within the confines of Port Eliot it is touching to see my husband try to keep the vibe alive and lose himself for a few hours, as far as is possible with me and the children in tow. On the second day he starts drinking at midday and doesn't stop. Six-year-old John keeps wanting to do handstands and needing things from the bag, but eventually Tom manages the impossible and breaks free.

He loves serendipitous encounters. Loads of his old friends are there and he makes some new ones. When we visit the stately home at the centre of the festival site, he jokes around with the elderly guides and charms them. He is the only person in that highly styled environment who looks like he just flew in from Ibiza, careering around in tattered shorts with a bottle of Prosecco in his pocket.

He keeps repeating the same thing over and over and laughing at his own jokes, like a drunken legionary from an Asterix book. I feel like I have lost him. This sometimes happens at home, and I always overreact. I'm scared of drunks because they seem like grotesque parodies of themselves – especially if, like Tom, they're usually more sensible than me. In retrospect his behaviour seems more endearing than sinister, but at the time I just felt abandoned, and terrified by the thought that I might have to be the one in charge if something bad happened. Whatever the context, wherever we are, whoever he's with, I need Tom to run like clockwork. He is my North Star and I am lost without him.

I didn't much feel like going back to Port Eliot – or indeed any festival – after that, so it became yet another little bit of the year that we'd spend apart. To raise my spirits while he was away I'd play rave music on Spotify, cranking up the volume and yearning to be back in the day. When people hear I was at university in 'Madchester' during the second summer of love, they invariably say, 'That must have been amazing', and I can practically see them forming a mental picture of me in flared jeans, dancing as if no one were looking to one of Graeme Park's twelve-hour sets. But I wasn't really there: I actually spent the second summer of love arguing with Labour modernisers and independents in the student union where I was women's officer, half a mile up the road from the Hacienda, where I was the women's officer. They were trying to reform the student union and my expense account was imperilled. I did take ecstasy a couple of times at 'the Hac' but found it utterly overwhelming in a far-from-'banging' way.

So my rave nostalgia is founded on a false memory, and this is the sort of thing that will most likely happen again and again as my past fades further and further from view. If my memory is unreliable, how can I find my way back to my biography? I long to smell and taste my childhood, or capture the essence of the era I grew up in, but all I can do is think about it. My previous attempt to write a memoir foundered because there was no evidence of my existence other than the ideas that had defined me. The polemical memoir should have been a good form for me, but I just corralled my experiences into an argument and the whole thing ended up as dry as dust.

This may have been because I was always too critical and analytical to really notice my own *mise en scène*. As a child I knew all about the anthropology of childhood, the sociology of childhood, the psychology of childhood; I read Peter and Iona Opie's *The Lore and Language of Schoolchildren* in the playground, and would spend hours analysing my peers and reflecting on the theory of being a child without ever putting any of it into practice. I read *The Drama of the Gifted Child* when I was eleven, but may just have taken it as a green light to carry on making a fuss about everything.

I do have one truly visceral childhood memory: being hurled to the ground and held there for the count of three in a game of British Bulldog. That alone tells you everything you need to know about growing up in the nasty, brutish 1970s. How many memories like that does it take to make a memoir? Will this process humanise my writing and make me more relatable? Bring my 'olden days' (as John calls them) back to life? Will you be able to smell the white dog shit and picture me in my Clothkits dungarees, a precocious and lonely figure dreaming of world domination? Will you *feel my pain*?

Recording my experiences has been surprisingly cathartic. The last time I kept a diary, I was a baby goth with a lighter fuel habit. My mother read it and threw a shoe at me; an understandable response. No more 'journaling' for me – but as a result I am now left with no notes, no recall, nothing to go on. Embarking on this memoir has been an act of faith.

We just got Anna a smartphone because she literally wouldn't stop asking, 'How will you know where I am if I don't have one?' Well, how did people manage before mobiles existed? My mother did worry when I was a teenager but basically knew I would always be in the graveyard on week nights and the same sweaty alternative nightclub – under Genghis Khan's Mongolian BBQ – on Fridays (you don't need a phone if you have a *scene*). I'm not sure that would have been enough for her if we'd been living in today's internet-enabled world, where keeping in touch with someone means not losing sight of them for even a fraction of a second – the temptation to constantly check on my whereabouts would have been too much. And we're all like that now, so it's almost impossible for anyone to get really lost.

I often got lost as a child because, with no smartphone or hi-vis jacket or wristband with my dad's phone number on, it was hard not to. When me and Dan were very young and our family still lived in London, Murph used to take us out every weekend. We'd go to Battersea Park's adventure playground, where no adults were allowed, and thence to the Asterix restaurant in King's Road or some Wimpy bar full of divorced fathers trying to impress their kids. But our favourite place was Hyde Park, which had the biggest slide in London (we called it the biggest slide in London but it may not have been and certainly wouldn't have impressed my children, who are jaded).

Murph had a rule for when people got lost: instead of looping around in circles and getting more lost, you had to go to the last place you saw him and wait. He also had a special whistle that was like a subdued version of Beethoven's Fifth: 'da-da-da dum'. If we heard it we would know he was near and try to follow the sound. These were sensible suggestions but it wasn't always easy to remember them in the heat of the moment.

Then, thrillingly, I got lost in Hyde Park. It was a novel experience and I wanted to prolong it. Instead of going to the last place I saw Murph or listening for his whistle, I turned off Bayswater Road into the park and ran along the shit-strewn paths towards the biggest slide in London. It was exhilarating; this was the only time in my life when getting lost meant breaking free and finding myself. I'd always been so attached to my mother but now, with the wind in my hair, I felt I could finally evade capture by that monster of inauthenticity and bring myself back to life. At the top of the slide I gazed down in triumph, only to see Murph waiting for me at the playground gates; he'd simply guessed where I would go and taken a short cut. It was galling indeed to reflect that my first bid for freedom had been foiled by my own bourgeois predictability.

It was a very different story when I lost Tom and the kids on the prom at Lyme Regis a few years ago. I went back to the last place I saw them, then realised I hadn't told them about Murph's law or the Mayday whistle. What hope did I have of finding them? I thought they would forget me and go back to the hotel to play croquet, and I would be left without my umbrella as the sky darkened and the storm clouds gathered.

I do seem to keep on losing people. I mislaid Murph when he married my stepmother; we didn't see much of him for years, and when we did it was awkward because Lottie wasn't great with my children. The conversation was stilted, and I thought Anna and John found her lack of animation disconcerting. But maybe I was just projecting.

My children lost their grandfather long before he died. In the old days he had been fully present, and more patient with them than me. He never got bored of the boring games – I can still see him and Anna in the garden, opening and closing the electric garage door again and again. The teddy bear he bought her is still on her bed.

As the disease progressed, though, he started to struggle with some of his grandfatherly duties and maintaining his benign countenance. There was a trace of tetchiness that may have been attributable to HD, though it's equally likely that he was just cross with me for not welcoming my new stepmother into the family. As far as I was concerned, my *froideur* was merely well-grounded resistance to an occupying force – within weeks of Lottie moving into the house I'd grown up in, the last remaining traces of Susan's presence had vanished as the decor changed beyond recognition. I felt like we didn't fit there any more. This probably would have happened whoever she had been, but the transition could have been handled with more sensitivity. We didn't visit much.

But at least he had someone to share his life with. He must have been lonely in that big house after Susan died, and Lottie's cooking was probably an improvement on the supermarket Cornish pasties he'd still have been living on otherwise.

Over the next few years his chorea inevitably worsened, and he had to give up both driving and reading. Eventually he decided (or was persuaded – I could never quite work out which) to start on an anti-chorea medication that stifled any urge to move so effectively that he couldn't even speak without considerable effort. But the pace of his mental degeneration remained slow and steady, so he was still completely compos mentis when he was moved into a care home in West Sussex.

The first time I went to visit him there, I was nervous about what I might find. And it wasn't just his well-being I was worried about – I couldn't help thinking that I myself might also end up in some variant of that home if/when I got too burdensome. (I do feel confident that Tom won't expel me from our house as long as I want to be there, but the cost of keeping me could prove ruinous. My hope is that I can carry on being looked after by carers with my family around me for as long as it's feasible; like Murph, I will need stimulation and love to make me feel alive when my brain cells are dying.)

Red Oaks was a large country house with beautiful manicured grounds but the lobby and sitting room were bland and boring, like a care home version of a Trust

House Forte hotel. If it had been me being sent there I would have been outraged by the aesthetic, but of course Murph wouldn't have cared about that. He would have cared about being patronised, though. Would they talk to him in a nursery school teacher's voice, assuming he couldn't understand what they were saying because he couldn't speak?

As care homes go, it was actually a pretty good one; it didn't look or feel institutional. But Murph didn't belong in a place that specialised in dementia. He had a nice enough room but confused old ladies were continually bursting into it. When we asked him what he thought of the place, he just said he was happy there. The wisdom of the decision to move him away from everything that was familiar could not be questioned. It would have stressed him out, which wouldn't have been good for him.

Murph's room was on the bottom floor, but where he really lived was in the parallel world of the rolling news channels. All day, every day it would be child abuse scandals, murders and the migrant crisis in pin-sharp high definition. I'm sure he was better informed than any of us, but possibly less relaxed. I used to take Anna and John to visit him every couple of months. He was always pleased to see them, even though it must have tired him out. He had never been very demonstrative but he'd hug me and hold on tight when we left. It was clear that he loved us as much as ever.

In HD, poignantly, love isn't one of the losses. Right up to the end, however it ends, people still feel profoundly connected to their friends and family. They miss them in the gaps between visits. When someone says they're going to visit and doesn't, this is a calamity and source of grief. Murph was always excited to see the children so it was sad when he was no longer able to hold their attention. They found his frozen face and halting speech disconcerting. John would do cartwheels rather than talk, and Anna struggled to maintain a one-sided conversation for longer than a minute or two. I got quite used to delivering my news as a monologue, but it was a lot to expect of them. When they said they didn't want to go any more, I couldn't really blame them. Murph's old business partner, Julian, started taking me instead. In the car on the way down he'd tell me funny stories about Murph's olden days.

Murph had always been very adaptable, so it's quite possible he adjusted to life in the home and didn't mind being stuck in his room 24/7. On the other hand, demotivation is one of the behavioural symptoms of HD. I'm sure the people at Red Oaks were respecting his wishes by leaving him pretty much to his own devices, but I thought they could have made more of an effort to find stimulating activities for him. Dan just hoped that the various drugs he was taking for the chorea tranquillised him sufficiently that he didn't care. He slept a lot, but did that mean he was zoned out and sedated or mentally there and bored out of his mind? It was hard to tell.

His condition deteriorated over years rather than days; there was a gradual ebbing away, with no dramatic scenes. Having refused to countenance a wheelchair for the first two years of his internment, we were all taken aback when he suddenly changed his mind and started asking to be wheeled along Brighton seafront. Dan used to drive him down there once or twice a week with 'Bat Out of Hell' blaring out of the stereo, and sometimes he'd even manage to sing along. I didn't notice when the slope of his decline steepened, possibly because I wanted him to carry on being my father in whatever diminished capacity. Then, one Friday in October, Dan called sounding worried: Murph was very ill with a stomach problem.

The problem was undiagnosed, and would remain so, because back when he was still healthy Murph had signed something that stipulated he was not to receive medical treatment if anything new should threaten his life after he'd already succumbed to the HD. A doctor had examined him but couldn't say for certain whether he had an ulcer or a tumour without taking him into hospital for tests, and that was out of the question. So nobody knew if this really was it or just a kind of awful dress rehearsal, but it clearly wasn't looking good.

My friend Decca swung into action, and there was a flurry of logistical arrangements that I was pleased for her to take charge of. We set off to Red Oaks at top speed, but it was the rush hour and the satnav kept sending us down twisty country lanes. When we finally got there after five hours on the road, we were told that Murph was getting worse. A horrible noise was coming from his room and I suddenly felt very scared. Forcing myself to go in, I was shocked to find him shaking and choreic, a total prisoner of HD for the first time – he hadn't been able to keep his usual medication down because he kept vomiting blood.

The one positive upshot of this was that he was much more able to talk than before, so it was almost like the old Murph had come back to us. He talked about his father's Cornish pasties and his grandchildren's achievements, and every so often, with enormous effort, made a joke. He kept saying he was worried about me, which he insisted was 'only natural'. When he asked Julian to look after me it felt like an emotionally binding promise which, when agreed, seemed to settle him for a couple of minutes – but as soon as I left the room he started asking Decca to pledge the same.

If I'm honest I was worried about me too, sick with fear that this scene would be repeated by a wretched, contorted future version of myself in another bed and a different room in who knew how many years' time. There was nothing anyone could do to stop this generational repeat, and no amount of money could ameliorate it – even with an upgrade, the genetic destination would be the same. I was witnessing what I would experience.

People came and went. We stayed overnight at a hotel and returned the next morning to find that Murph's condition had unexpectedly improved – he was out of bed and keeping down both food and meds. The doctor felt that he was probably out of the woods, although there was obviously no way to be certain, and Murph himself seemed understandably keen to be left alone after three solid days of being wept at. Baffled but relieved, we drove back to London. And Murph died.

The people at Red Oaks said that it had been too sudden for him to have suffered much, and that someone had been with him when it happened. I wanted to believe them but instinctively felt that if he'd actually died alone in screaming agony, this was not something they'd be likely to tell us. I wish I could say he was at peace in that last weekend of his life, but it wasn't just the HD that was agitating him – as I was to discover later, he was also feeling guilty about what awaited me and Dan after he was gone.

Lottie said, 'He would want us to give him a good send-off', which was hard to argue with even if it meant a truce until after the funeral. Dan and I started collaborating on a eulogy, Lottie was in charge of the order of service and her son from her previous marriage would be choosing the music, in consultation with us. Hamish is a good man who genuinely loved Murph but he just couldn't get his head around the idea of Meat Loaf at a funeral; I know Dan suggested it to him more than once, but every time he'd just smile enigmatically and say it was okay, he had a few ideas.

The funeral is a bit of a blur. The order of service's front cover had small mistakes that irritated me enormously. 'A celebration for the life of Vivian Foster Raven' – but it should have been 'of', not 'for', and 'Murph', not 'Vivian'. We did get 'Bat Out of Hell' at the start of the service but the 'music for reflection' turned out to be Eric Clapton's 'Tears in Heaven', a turgid ditty whose admitted appropriateness for the occasion was somewhat undermined by the fact that Lottie had also insisted on having it played at her and Murph's wedding several years earlier.

But the worst was yet to come: when the curtains closed for the committal, on went Elton John's 'Rocket Man'. What was Hamish thinking? How could we cry to that? I realise it must have been a tough call as, apart from Meat Loaf, Murph had only ever liked 'Hallelujah Chorus' and The Swingle Singers, but he certainly wasn't an Elton John fan – and even if he had been, that still wouldn't have been the right song! I started to think about how furious Susan would have been with this MOR choice … and then I started to smile, because it struck me that this was exactly the sort of thing Murph might have done to annoy her and/or me back in the day. He might not have planned it himself, but he was having the last laugh.

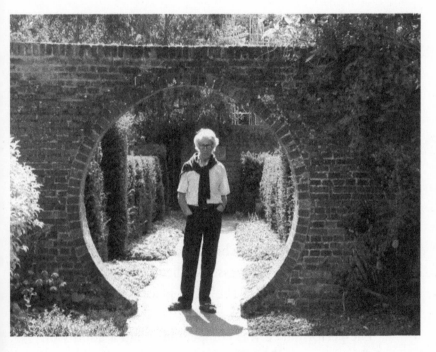

The last photo of Murph

4

Empathy

Kae Tempest is a poet and rapper who shares my doomy worldview but expresses it better than I ever could, with poems and songs about the lives of ordinary people that are unapologetically political and full of what contemporary commentators like to call 'radical empathy'. I took Tom to see Kae at the Brixton Academy.

I'd been counting down the days; I hadn't felt like this about a performer since Paul Weller in the 80s. My passion for him had been inscribed in blood when, bored in a biology lesson, I'd scratched 'The Jam' into my forearm with the point of a compass. I wished I could fashion my own 'Kae T' tattoos in the same place while watching TV but feared the repercussions.

The performance was compelling. I had a good view of the stage, and Kae's charisma carried us all away. All but one of us, that is – on the pavement outside the venue, Tom shocked me by saying that all the 'polemicising' had left him cold, and that the poem about PTSD had reminded him of one of *Private Eye*'s Harold Pinter parodies. He felt that the poetry *lacked* poetry. I could see what he meant, but at the same time it felt like he was attacking me. I am very sensitive; I have visions that stop me from sleeping. But I haven't found a way to make my sensitivity relatable. It irritates Tom when I go on about Vladimir Putin and North Korea's hydrogen bomb. Inspired by Kae, I tried to write poetry but it didn't work. I may be too old to rap.

We went to a curry house near Euston and Tom drank more pints. He had something important to communicate to me, something he'd said before but never with such conviction: 'You empathise with the migrants dying in the Med, the homeless man camped outside the betting shop on the high street, swindled pensioners on *Rogue Traders*, puppies and terrorists – but you don't empathise with me. Or the children! You're a tyrant at home, preoccupied with whatever is in your head, and you never really listen to any of us.'

When we got home he said the same thing again in different words, about fourteen times, before falling asleep on the sofa bed. I stayed awake, replaying all the times I had pounced on him the minute he came home from work and asked him to sort out my computer issues, resolve my work dilemmas, cook my tea or iron my dress. I felt so sorry and guilty. My inhumanity may have been caused by my upbringing or HD but, wherever it had come from, I had to take responsibility for it. If I couldn't change the way I was – and I had tried – I at least needed to think about how I could lessen its impact on others.

I looked miserable the next morning. Anna sensed that something was wrong.

'How was it, then? You look tired.'

'Amazing! She is a secular preacher. Do you know what "secular" means?'

'No. Ring her up, Mum! Invite her round for tea! I'd love to see her again.'

Because, yes, I'd actually *met* Kate T in the early days of my feminist publishing project, which started as an attempt to relaunch *Spare Rib* with no ads or puff pieces. I wanted to create a platform for divergent voices, where all opinions would be equally respected. It was a tall order; feminists were so used to slagging each other off that the idea of a broad church where you had to empathise with those you disagreed with was radical indeed. Would it be possible to have a women's magazine that wasn't snarky? Kate came to one of our focus groups and everyone fell in love with her, including my daughter. Anna was in charge of the whiteboard and keeping the discussion on topic, which would have been a tough job even for someone who wasn't a nine-year-old. Kate was warmly appreciative of her efforts and never talked down to her.

I often asked myself, 'What would Kate do?' in the dark days that were to follow, as I clashed with the founders of the original *Spare Rib* over my plan to use the name. Anna, who was reading Harry Potter at the time, had nicknames for Rosie Boycott and Marsha Rowe that I *might* have used myself, I'm ashamed to say ... Does radical empathy extend to Lord Voldemort and Draco Malfoy?

*

After Tom's talk I was acutely aware of my empathy levels and kept gauging them while watching the news and, more importantly, when the kids came home from school. Loss of empathy is one of the most challenging emotional elements of HD.

People with Huntington's disease may sometimes seem self-centred, uncaring and thoughtless. Their apparent disregard for the emotional needs of a partner can be hurtful, and is especially poignant when it contrasts with a formerly loving and caring relationship; the natural tendency is for the partner to feel personally slighted. In these situations, the person with HD is not being deliberately awkward, wilful or unkind – their apparent self-centredness is a consequence of the loss of mental flexibility associated with Huntington's disease. Individuals may no longer be able to put themselves in another person's shoes or weigh up both sides of an argument. They may genuinely fail to see how their remarks or actions affect others.

The disease can also impair a person's ability to experience the complex range of subtle emotions that contribute to interpersonal relationships, so that their emotions become shallow or 'blunted'. The adverse effect of HD on an individual's capacity for sympathy and empathy is yet another reason why it can have such a devastating impact on families.

My various impairments stopped our household running smoothly until we found a carer, Ade. She also helped with admin and my to-do list. But empathy can't be outsourced; my young family needed a mother who could connect with them and I was often too self-absorbed, thinking about the holes in my slippers, my next feminist project or this book.

Tom parented for the two of us (as well as earning all the money). He remembered their PE kit, involves them in creative activities like baking so they don't sit in front of the telly all day, controlled their texting and took Anna to football on Saturdays. More importantly, he was there for them emotionally when I was distracted and semi-detached. I forgot lots of things, so couldn't be trusted with their weekly schedule. I even forgot John's Christmas show ('You were the only mummy who wasn't there. The *only mummy*!').

If I feel guilty about the Christmas show, there must be hope for me. Could I have spent so long brooding about my inhumanity if I really *was* inhumane? I've read accounts of HD sufferers who feel no shame about behaving inappropriately or splashing out on cars they can't afford, whereas I am constantly wracked with guilt about ill-advised purchases and being a shit parent. I welcome this in, as a sign of life.

Tom has good reason to believe I was prematurely unempathic. Our relationship wasn't loving or collaborative in the first place, so there were few reserves of goodwill to draw on when HD came to call. The early years of our marriage were like our wedding, but this time it wasn't Murph who was paying. I got Tom to pay for childcare because I wanted to talk to Anna and John, not cook for them or clean up after them. Before they could talk I found them boring and irritating. Feeling personally slighted by their demands, I'd long for a Mary Poppins to descend from the sky and rescue me. I argued Tom into finding an agency nanny – she might have cost the earth, but who could put a price on my freedom of expression and peace of mind? I had never been a huge fan of babies anyway, but this felt like something else – postnatal depression, resentment at being upstaged or a combination of the two.

This isn't easy to admit, but I felt they were stealing the limelight. However sleep deprived, Tom seemed to find them enchanting, while I fantasised about imposing a famously illiberal regime of baby training recommended by a working mother friend – just leave them to cry, just for a few minutes ... ! – which I knew he'd be against. I found it hard to concentrate on my writing even with the nanny, so I lobbied Tom for a garden office. When he had paid for that, I used it for a couple of weeks and then asked for it to be soundproofed because the noises from the street were too distracting.

I never had a 'proper' job (even the *Modern Review* had hardly been 9–5) because I couldn't stand anyone telling me what to do; my idea of independence was all about intellectual freedom, not paying my way. We had a joint account that I thought of as a temporary loan from Tom while I worked out how to earn money for clothes and childcare without selling out. I never checked the balance because I was convinced that the moment when I would be able to put in as much as I was taking out was just around the corner – and at least I'd stopped getting taxis everywhere, right ... ?

For some reason I believed that my views would still be as marketable as they had been in the past, and I was encouraged by the relative ease of a crowdfunding campaign for our now-nameless feminist project. We raised a lot of money in just a few days, which seemed to confirm that the model we had arrived at – a website funded by members paying a monthly subscription – would be workable and sustainable. It also suggested a pressing need for an intelligent women's magazine that didn't patronise its readers. When the news of what we were planning leaked to the press, we were overwhelmed by goodwill and offers of help. The long-awaited feminist uprising felt close at hand.

Because we wanted to operate from the outset as an ethical, anti-capitalist enterprise, it was very important to me that we paid our writers and editors properly. So many other publications were run by unpaid interns – posh graduates, in other words – and I didn't want ours to stumble on the same hurdle of accessibility. But did I treat my husband as respectfully as the people working with me? Reader, I did not. If anything, my demands on him grew, in both frequency and volume, because my ability/inclination to take care of the domestic stuff had fled further than ever. The project may have been going well but there was nothing left of me for my family.

The pantry moths that had taken over our kitchen were thriving (a grim metaphor for my emotional slovenliness!) because I never had time to look in the cupboards or close the cereal boxes or put lids on honey jars. There were things in the kitchen cupboard that were years out of date and open packets everywhere. Poor John found a maggot in one of his organic cereal bars, which made him cry. This should have been a warning to me to change my behaviour, but instead of putting everything in Tupperware and commencing a lengthy war of attrition against the pests (as Tom advised), I called Rentokil. They gave me a quote of £800 and I told them to go ahead, even though they couldn't promise it would actually work.

It never occurred to me to ask Tom if he minded living in a Jan Švankmajer film because his unfailing good humour always made him look like he was enjoying himself, but in fact I was draining his inner resources. When I got the feminist website – now called *Feminist Times* – off the ground, our kitchen table became its base of operations and Tom was around all the time, contributing to our discussions about gender politics. Instead of being asked about his day when he came home from work he'd be confronted with a tangle of personal and political dilemmas which, by virtue of his sex, he was ill equipped to unravel. He cooked delicious meals for all the feminists, then put the children to bed while I had boozy discussions about sexism and transgender rights long into the night. The irony of having such a benign and consistent man at the tiller while I spent so much of my time complaining about men was lost on me.

Should I blame my upbringing for my lack of empathy and tendency to subtly bully people? The child-centred parenting model that Susan followed was based on the idea that children should set their own rules, which obviously makes for short-term harmony but also means that all the little courtesies that show you are thinking of other people – those small but important indications of empathy – go unlearned. Susan thought table manners were bourgeois, so I grew up speaking with my mouth full and didn't manage to break the habit until I was about forty.

As a teenager, I thought I was special and Dan wasn't. He didn't seem to care that much but it was depressing to think of him mooching around in his bedroom the whole time, failing to be impressed by me. To cheer him up I gave him a horrible-looking fish from my old aquarium, the bottom-feeding loach. The aquarium had once been full of beautiful tropical fish, but these had all been electrocuted when I smashed the heater against the glass. The bottom-feeding loach was the only survivor, a revolting specimen that was clearly the cockroach of fishes. It managed to live for another five years in Dan's room – a record for my childhood pets, which never lasted long.

I also feel remorse for the way I treated my guinea pigs, who were kept in hutches in the basement with nowhere to run around. Sarah and Louise were out of sight, out of mind, just like Dan (and whatever the fish was called). It may be too late to apologise to my neglected pets but I have at least said sorry to Dan. Fortunately, he has just about survived growing up with me.

Susan constantly reminded me that failure to fulfil my potential would be a fate worse than death. When I did really badly in my O levels she tried to get me back in line for greatness by reminding me what was at stake: 'You're going to be someone, don't fuck it up.' This quote from my first boyfriend had really impressed her and she wanted me to keep it in mind, so she made a sign and stuck it on my bedroom wall. But Dave Copping's words were uninspiring and enervating. From that day to this I have been burdened with both a sense of entitlement and *a terror of fucking it up* that have made me a narcissistic perfectionist who, paradoxically, can take no pleasure in her achievements.

Years later, when I was married to Tom, I tried to write a book about narcissism in my expensive writing hut away from the rattle and hum of family life, but it just felt a bit ... narcissistic. It took me ten years to reach this conclusion, with Tom supporting me financially and emotionally throughout. When I should have been writing, I found myself 'hate reading' a number of fellow narcissists' blogs.

I hated them because they were less self-aware than me but more successful. A middle-class journalist who became the editor of a society paper and then married a lord blogged about the bluebells in the garden of her stately home; I knew more about her life than I did about Anna and John's. An English woman living in France blogged about her affair with a married man, and actually got it made into a book. And then there was that feminist fashion blog by that other hack who really annoyed me ... Why do I find these people so fascinating? I've often asked myself this question. Am I projecting my own narcissism onto them? Are they the innocent victims of my psychological manoeuvring?

Tom says I grew out of narcissism, as he'd hoped I would. After I stopped working on my book but before the HD diagnosis, I had a little window of humanity in which we got on fantastically well. I would ask him about his life and, more importantly, listen to the answers. 'How was your day, darling?' 'Are you going out? Have fun! I won't wait up.' I felt like I was getting to know him for the first time. Now that I'd stopped behaving like a child, we were able to discuss things like adults.

Suddenly Tom was doing things because he wanted to, not because he felt he had to. His friends came over and they were all fascinating; I found everything interesting when I was paying attention, and my life felt richer as a result. I even managed to visit Tom's family's holiday home in Dorset without moaning about the cold. With our relationship properly balanced, I felt it might be possible to repair the damage of my narcissism. For the first time in my life I was enjoying myself without drowning anyone else out. As a symbol of this new dawn, I stopped raiding our joint account and we had a plan for paying off our debts.

It didn't last. Fast-forward a couple of years and I was finishing the milk before the others could get to it and sending Tom to the shop to buy more – every single morning. I never slept and made sure no one else did. My needs blotted out everyone else's, and when I wanted something I had to have it NOW. I was always pestering

Tom to have sex with me, and never took no for an answer. I needed to be fed, loved and listened to before the children, which was a tall order as I had never been more unlovable. The relatives of people with HD are asked to perform a feat of empathy; we demand love with childish persistence, needing it for validation and reassurance of our humanity, while behaving in an alienating way. My lack of empathy delivered a mortal blow to my marriage.

To begin with, we didn't realise that my behaviour could have been caused by HD – it just felt like I was reverting to form, a selfish bully again, stealing everyone's air. Instead of changing me beyond recognition, the disease was turning me into an amplified version of my old self. But the fact that it wasn't my fault this time probably wouldn't have been much comfort to Tom anyway. He wasn't very kind to me, which was understandable. He'd drink a bottle of wine every night and we'd argue until dawn.

Annoyingly, it turns out that Buddha thought of radical empathy before me and Kate T! I discovered this at a meditation retreat in Devon. 'Metta' means unconditional love for all beings. We tried to cultivate it during meditation by visualising people from our lives and showering them with metta. I found it easier to send benevolent thoughts to the man behind the counter in the organic shop than to my husband, but the coordinators assured me I was on the right track; it takes a lot of practice to direct metta to all beings. I took up meditation in the hope that it would train me to empathise with my family. I was still in a world of my own, but at least I was starting to think about other people's needs.

The day before one of Tom's work trips was always a blur of activity, so it didn't seem all that surprising when he took all the rubbish from our junkyard of a garden to the dump in a hired van. He had fixed the drains, called the gas people about the leak, taken John to his trapeze lesson, mowed the lawn, batch-cooked for the week, hung up all the washing and made daily to-do lists so none of us could forget anything while he was away, including a detailed breakdown of packed lunches, the kit list for John's school camp and reminders to water the garden. After a few days it occurred to me that this may have been a dress rehearsal for when he left for good, and so it proved.

We had agreed to live apart. Tom deserved a second chance to be intimate with someone who was still capable of intimacy. It wasn't just that, though – as well as desexualising me, HD has blunted my emotions. I hardly ever cry, and I sense that my emotional range is not the same as other people's. When I told someone at a party that my frozen face didn't mean I was unenthusiastic about meeting them, they said I smiled with my eyes.

Tom promised he would make sure I had enough support, and he has been true to his word, but having people around to help with the practicalities and keep me company in the evenings is not the same as having a husband. For months I was consumed with regret about taking him for granted when I should have been cherishing him. He seemed heroic to me now that I could see him properly, and the more I empathised with him, the more in love with him I felt. After years of slamming doors in his face, I wanted to open one for him.

We made a plan for how we were going to tell the children we were separating, but I ended up ignoring it – I'd always tried to be straightforward with them and felt I needed to account for the fact that I was gloomier than usual. Anna barely looked up from her phone: 'It was pretty obvious, Mum. He was living on a houseboat for three months.' She also pointed out that he had spent the last two years camped out in the worst room in the house, a poorly constructed extension that is too hot in summer and too cold in winter. His IKEA wardrobe was falling apart and the Wi-Fi signal was weak, so he couldn't watch the things he needed to for work. Anna said she wanted to live with me and seemed pleased that Tom and I were getting on, unlike her best friend's divorced parents who couldn't be in the same room as each other.

John is very sensitive, so I was sad but not surprised when he told me how affected he had been by his parents' rows: 'You thought I was upstairs when you were shouting at Dad, but I was outside the door.' Then, on our way back from school one day, he said, 'If you and Dad divorced, it would mean a Huntington's lady would be on her own.' Me and Anna reassured him that Tom would always look after me even if we were no longer living together, but of course he was still worried. 'Can children get Huntington's? Does my worrying mean I have it?' We found a link to the Huntington's Disease Youth Organisation website, but Anna said she hated the colours and found the tone patronising.

As for me, I was heartbroken and sometimes indignant. How the hell could he leave me when, in spite of the illness, my behaviour had never been more reasonable? Deep down, though, I realised that if I'd treated him better before I got ill then we'd still have been together. He may only have stuck with me for as long as he did because his parents had brought him up to be dutiful to the point of self-abasement – if it hadn't been for the HD, he would probably have left me years ago.

Now that I didn't want to talk about it, everyone seemed to be asking me about our wedding. John even boasted about it to a friend's mother on a playdate: 'Mum and Dad's wedding was so "extra". They stopped the traffic in Brighton! I wish I could have been there.' With every retelling it would become a little more extravagant, and I would have a little more time to reflect on what an awful false start it had been for our marriage. I found myself feeling quite guilty about it. 'Extra' means over the top, and it's hard to disagree with that assessment. When Tom left, I thought about whether I should leave the wedding pictures on the mantelpiece or put them away somewhere. Then I had a proper look at them – at Decca in that awful dress I made her wear and Tom in his slightly-too-big Austin Reed suit – and was so charmed that I decided to leave them where they were.

When Tom moved into a flat around the corner in 2018, we still had a good time together and stayed up all night talking every so often; confusingly, we had never got on better. He said letting him go had been an act of love that would be an inspiration for Anna and John in years to come. It was always horrible when he went home to his flat, though. I couldn't stand the idea of him being with someone else, not least because they would have had to be unusually intelligent and empathic to get their heads around our unconventional set-up – a woman of substance, in other words, who felt like competition when I contemplated her. Then I started to get used to it. The only thing to do is to accept the new normal. I wish I'd nurtured him when I had the chance, but it's too late for regret. I don't want to feel burdened with guilt about the times I forgot his birthday, and can see only one way of avoiding this: *remember it from now on*. I want to celebrate the good things we still have.

John empathises with me, picking things up when I drop them (although, sadly, he must still be paid to embark on any household chore that takes longer than three minutes). Anna and Tom and even Tom's family empathise with me, offering constant reassurance that none of this is my fault. Somehow, though, I can't now seem to empathise with myself. My therapist kept crying when I told her about the end of my marriage and the daily frustrations of life with HD, but I didn't. I could see that it was right to work on surmounting my guilt, but forgiveness and self-acceptance seemed elusive.

When everything had settled down, though, I started to think I hadn't done such a bad job, given the hand I'd been dealt. I'd helped to look after my family and kept it on an even keel in demanding circumstances without moaning or longing to be back at the top of the bill. I found this unexpectedly rewarding and did not experience motherhood as a demotion, as I might once have done. We bought John a hamster, which he called Plain Jane Mary Lou Raven (all our pets have been Ravens in the interests of fairness, because Anna and John are both Sheahans like Tom). John started playing a range of instruments without needing to be chivvied to practise for exams. I started writing in the study next to the kitchen, and discovered that I didn't really mind the noise of the children coming in and out with their friends after all. We were committed to making the house a hub of creativity where everyone is nurtured and supported, and that's what it has become.

5
Madness

'You're weird, Mum.'

The kids are always saying this and they are right. I play weird games with them. I hated board games even before I had HD, but now the rules of Labyrinth and Scrabble are impenetrable. They all want me to play Twister because I'm precarious and easy to topple. Dan gave us a Wii, thinking I would enjoy Super Mario Galaxy and that it would be something for me to do in the evenings instead of watching telly. The graphics are beautiful but I can't use the joystick. I always press too hard and Mario just careers around his world like a sailor on shore leave.

Imaginative games peopled by strange characters are my stock-in-trade. I routinely ventriloquise our cat Archie, a toy cat called Mary Lou (John named the hamster after her), the ducks in the bath and all the characters in our games. It's always the same voice, whether I'm playing a horse or a bank clerk. 'Play horseys,' John commands. I am always the horse and he is perched uncomfortably on my back. Now he's bigger it's getting harder, but the voice is still easy to find. We take trips to horsey-land, a horse version of Disneyland where we stay in a nice hotel and eat granola bars and quince. When people visit he tries to get me to 'do the voice'. 'What voice?' '*The* voice, the one you always do!'

But of course I do all sorts of voices these days, if you count the involuntary vocalisations. I make strange sing-songy sounds on the stairs and weird noises when I'm watching the news. Anna says she finds them comforting but I'm starting to feel like the crazy cat lady from *The Simpsons*.

Only a small proportion of HD sufferers experience schizophrenia-like symptoms such as delusions and hallucinations, but we all share a propensity for incandescent rage. I've flown off the handle regularly and our poor house bears the scars. I once bashed my head against the radiator in the kitchen and pulled it off the wall. It's so upsetting to keep losing things, and I'm also angry with everyone else for not helping me keep track of things or looking for them when I lose them.

When Tom and I used to argue, I'd scream like a soap opera character and throw things at him; all of our wedding-list crockery was sacrificed to HD. Our living-room door has been kicked repeatedly, scaring the children. If anything went wrong while he was away, which it always seemed to, my anxiety would be supplanted by white-hot fury. Many domestic crises have been exacerbated by my response, but fortunately Anna is always calm and collected. Tom was in Outer Mongolia when a fault with the washing machine fused all our lights, but Anna worked through the problem with a friend on the phone and even took the clothes to the laundrette. She helps with my computer and mobile phone issues, and my dumb resistance to finding out how to work our 'smart' TV.

And at least we don't have to live in some sleepy village where my eccentricity would be the talk of the local pub – the madder I get in Kentish Town, the more I fit in. I don't know if my neighbourhood has more eccentrics than most, but it certainly feels that way. The high street is like an Alexander McQueen catwalk, full of disturbing characters. A Victorian lady in a full-length bustle skirt and straw boater passes our window every morning, presumably on her way to work. I wonder what happens when she gets there. Does she fold her Victoriana away and reach for the modern dress? She carries a book but no purse or mobile phone, eschewing the trappings of the twenty-first century. No half measures; her character is fully realised. She seems bad tempered, as if en route to a particularly tiresome 'at home', and her manner discourages potential enquiries.

The doll lady can be found in the local Cancer Research shop, buying clothes for her babies. The staff are on hand to help this harassed mother of ten find something suitable among the babygros. In her old-fashioned pram there are ten baby dolls. In her head they are screaming blue murder. What happens when she gets home? It must take forever to feed them all. Do they need an afternoon nap?

The angry lady's bright red cheeks are evidence of her literal-mindedness. They've just started anger management courses at the women's health centre in Camden, but the angry lady clearly hasn't attended; she is shouting the odds and berating the sky. The red make-up smeared across her cheeks is not rouge but something raw and real, like a bruised cherry. I want to buy some to put in my bottom drawer, for when my illness is more advanced. The original angry lady might get annoyed with me for stealing her shtick but I will personalise the act and make it my own: the angry Raven kicking off in the post office queue, frightening the children with her weird noises and scrounging fags off the teenagers. My tattered Primark dress will be accessorised with a tattoo of a Raven eating a skull: my state of mind reified.

My history of mental illness has segued so seamlessly into HD that it's hard to say where one ended and the other began, but I can't help wondering now whether my genes were to blame for the breakdown I had in the 90s.

I was being paid a fortune to write my column while living rent-free in West Kensington, and had nothing to spend it on apart from drugs and clothes. I never took public transport or paid for my own lunch – bliss was it in that dawn to be a young mediawhore. I didn't realise how lucky I was or think for a moment that the generation after me would struggle to make a living from journalism and have to construct portfolio lives to fund their writing.

Susan was pleased to see me established as a journalist, and disinclined to register the psychological cost of my staying there. Column day was always stressful. I had no idea how to structure a piece and couldn't draft one either. Everyone kept telling me to draft them but I couldn't. I wanted them to be perfect – the idea of a 'good enough' column didn't fit with my Atlantic Bar persona or Dave Copping's motivational prophecy. With a deadline looming I'd go into meltdown and ring Susan in hysterics, asking her to write my intro. This happened every week, and I'd miss my deadline every time. I couldn't work out what was wrong with me.

I saw Oasis at Maine Road in Manchester in 1996 when they were in their pomp, and for the first time in my life it felt like I was in the right place at the right time. Embarrassing to relate, but I had an elaborate fantasy world back then which enabled me to both shag Liam Gallagher and cast my rivals into a 90s version of purgatory, with Geri Halliwell officiating. The drugs *did* work – that was the problem. I was becoming more and more detached from reality and the writer's block was getting worse. Susan was really worried, but I self-diagnosed and managed to persuade a private psychiatrist to agree that I had attention deficit disorder.

I was on Ritalin when I wrote the proposal for my feminist advice book, and it was a wonderfully prolific period. In the long wakeful nights I'd turn out op-ed pieces by the dozen, sex pieces for *Cosmo* and reams of contentious cultural commentary, but I couldn't sleep or eat – I was just about managing to consume one tin of Dunn's River Nurishment a day. I went back to the doctor and he gave me diazepam, along with some temazepam to take the edge off. Rather than face the fact that I was going slowly mad, I continued to diagnose myself with a different syndrome every day.

I had picked up a very unpleasant on/off boyfriend along the way who'd convinced me that I was a terrible person because I didn't want to hang out with his family. He was the original toxic bachelor, luring women to their doom. We argued all the time and I always came off worse.

His world was immaculate: the bijou townhouse, the vintage car, the exquisitely manicured fingernails. In a desperate bid to win his approval I bought the women's version of his watch, a Saab convertible and a flat in Kentish Town – but I kept spilling Diet Coke on his sofa, and felt messy and unkempt on his arm. A passer-by once found me weeping on the street near his house.

This relationship nearly finished me off. Poor Susan was beside herself with worry. I crashed and realised, belatedly, that I needed help; my mad friend Derek booked me into The Priory.

I had, of course, been looking forward to seeing Robbie Williams in a straitjacket or Kate Moss rocking a Napoleon hat but, sadly, my stay did not turn out to coincide with any major celebrity breakdowns. There were other consolations, though: I tend to like institutions anyway, and this one felt so much like my secondary school that I started to feel comfortable there quite quickly. Criticising the regime gave me a renewed sense of purpose and I enjoyed hanging out with the patients, stirring things up and giving them advice about their problems (which I still, inexplicably, felt qualified to do).

There was a charismatic psychiatrist there who all the women were in love with, Massimo Riccio. He weaned me off the pills I'd got from the Harley Street doctor, with a lot of tutting about how I'd been misdiagnosed. After a couple of weeks' detoxing he put me on Prozac, which was a new drug at the time.

Susan used to come and get my washing at the end of every week, but I was distant with her – I was starting to realise that the lack of boundaries in our relationship might have contributed to my breakdown, and there was a lot to untangle. But I was also, frankly, undergoing a massive comedown from all the recreational drugs I'd been taking, and I could hardly blame her for that. So in that sense the comedown became a moment of insight for me, when I started to see things as they really were; I was beginning to understand that my ups and downs could take a toll on the people close to me.

Many HD sufferers experience depression, and it's at its worst at the beginning of the illness and the end. There is a lull in the middle. When I think back to the time when I was most depressed, I picture myself fighting with both my husband and my hair; I had a high-maintenance bob which defined me, or so I thought. When things started falling apart after my diagnosis I became ever more invested in my hair but also less able to perform the complex ritual of straightening it, which required three mirrors positioned at very particular angles and just the right amount of Moroccan oil.

I was very isolated in this era. We'd have people round for dinner every now and then but it never really worked. On one occasion I brought my hairdryer, mirrors and straighteners to the table with me. As soon as the conversation started, I turned on the hairdryer and drowned it out. Our guest was an old friend I hadn't seen in years, and I was wearing a tunic dress that was far too short for me. I still feel embarrassed when I conjure this scene.

Like the angry lady's cheeks, my hair was a signifier of my inner turmoil. I was mortally terrified of facing the encroaching darkness with no support, because I'd burned my bridges and alienated my husband just when I needed him most – but, paradoxically, that only seemed to make my behaviour worse. We were in debt because of the money I'd frittered away on fripperies. The Vola taps were always mentioned, and my expensive haircuts. And sex, why was I always pestering him about sex? Couldn't I see what was happening? The more I went on about it the less attractive I became, but I couldn't stop. We argued every day and most of the night. His retreat to the sofa bed was traumatic but completely understandable.

The weekends were the worst. I'd be tormented by restlessness for most of the night and kept on getting up for bowls of cereal, like I did when I was pregnant. On Saturday mornings I would sit in the leather chair in the kitchen, bewailing my lot and demanding poached eggs. My life was over and I might as well just accept that. My career had stalled while Tom kept winning prizes for his work, and my two young children were clearly to blame, even though I didn't look after them. At that point I was still in denial about the depression and didn't attribute it to HD, perceiving my low mood to be a well-judged response to the fact that my life was shit. I was a bit young to be having a mid-life crisis, though.

Our house, with its vertiginous stairwell and over-abundance of dark corners, was the perfect setting for a Gothic novel that was inappropriate for children. Aggressive, miserable and unmedicated, I was both haunter and haunted. It all came to a head one stormy night when, pursued by demons, I punched out the window on the second-floor landing.

I can see now that I wasn't responsible for my actions, but at the time the attribution was difficult. More than anything else, I wanted Tom to be kind to me. It had the opposite effect, though. He was angry when I got him out of bed to patch me up, a first-aider without compassion, applying pressure to the wounds to staunch the flow of blood and then putting plasters on with cold efficiency, as if I were attention-seeking and he were the victim, not me. Perhaps he was right. My knuckles were swollen for weeks but the feeling of being judged by him lasted longer.

I suggested marriage therapy and he reluctantly agreed. The Tavistock Centre is where North London marriages have been going to die since 1948, so I was at least reasonably confident that we wouldn't be the worst thing they'd ever seen. The waiting room was full of middle-class people raking over the coals and longing for an exit route that wouldn't hurt the children.

Our sessions used to start at eight o'clock in the morning, which meant negotiating the Tube in the rush hour, so I was always late. The therapist was an immaculate (they always are) woman with a neat bob. How did she get it like that? I was fascinated. We argued about the same things in the same tones of voice as we did at home, with the therapist as an expensive witness trying to find common ground. Looking back, I wish someone had told me to see a psychiatrist before embarking on marriage guidance therapy. In my state of mind, it was the wrong tool for the job – if anything, it only made matters worse.

The therapist's verdict? 'I think you're *both* depressed.'

We argued in the street outside, and I grabbed Tom's bike because I didn't want him to go to work until he'd accepted his part in our downfall. I kept saying I was sorry and I really was, but couldn't work out how to stop this cycle of selfishness and self-recrimination. And I was disinhibited, another HD trait, which meant I didn't mind arguing in front of the children. I'd even follow Tom up the road in my dressing gown when he was taking them to school, oblivious to the twitching curtains and too self-absorbed to notice the looks on their faces. The effect of HD on family life is immeasurable. I tried to explain it to Anna, and I think she was old enough to understand – but she did say she *would* be cross with me for being cross all the time, if she didn't know about my illness.

I thought about suicide but couldn't decide how to do it. Murph had always said he would throw himself off Beachy Head when the time came but never got around to it. In his later years other people made decisions on his behalf, keeping him ticking over even though his quality of life was poor. If his former self, the Murph of our childhood, could have seen the person stuck in front of the TV at Red Oaks, unable to speak for years, would he have expedited the cliff-edge plan, knowing that he would lack the will and wherewithal to carry it out in the future? He'd kept on saying he was happy there, but only to avoid controversy. The time had come and gone for him.

I too considered Beachy Head – in fact, I only really dropped the idea because I didn't fancy being accosted by one of the Christians who patrol those cliffs nowadays, trying to convince lost souls that human life is sacred. When I mentioned this to someone at the complex depression and trauma unit in Camden, they booked me in to see a psychiatrist that same week. The psychiatrist gave me a combination of antidepressants and mood stabilisers, and twenty free sessions with a psychologist.

I'd already been in therapy on and off for years. I enjoyed analysing my problems and entertaining therapists, although the good ones usually saw through this strategy and seemed (or were) impervious to my charms. My last therapist, Adele, had never given me any advice, and I'd never even known if she was smiling at my stories as I lay on her couch in West Hampstead, free-associating into space. Carly was less rigorous and daunting, more like a wise friend who empathised with me and offered helpful suggestions about how to change the dynamic with Tom.

After a few sessions, and before I had time to object, I was edged into mindfulness-based CBT. As well as arguing about money and parenting, Tom and I were now arguing about therapeutic modalities. He approved of CBT but I thought its focus on transforming negative automatic thoughts set people up to fail (when you couldn't get rid of them you blamed yourself, not your therapist or CBT), and its one-size-fits-all approach ignored unconscious motivations for feeling and thoughts, reducing our beautiful minds to equations on a whiteboard.

Wisely, Carly emphasised the meditation and mindfulness elements, which did make sense to me – all the evidence suggests that meditation works better than antidepressants for some people. But it was a tricky thing to master when all I really wanted was a quick fix. In the 'breathing space' at the beginning of each session I would think about Carly's dip-dyed hair and wonder how much it had cost. The room was always either overheated or freezing cold as we talked about the here and now, and made plans for a future me beyond this current crisis that seemed eminently achievable until I stepped outside.

I started writing an article for the *Guardian* that looked at the arguments for and against voluntary euthanasia. I wanted to call it 'The Allure of Suicide' but I'm fairly sure they didn't go with that. For research purposes I spent several months coolly surveying my options and trying different suicide scenarios on for size. I assumed Dignitas wouldn't take me because I wouldn't be ill enough to qualify – and if I waited until I was, I could be suffering terribly for years. Alternatively, I could book into the Chelsea Hotel in New York (which apparently is still there, but more like a tribute to itself than an authentic bohemian hangout) and take some Nembutal with me. Nembutal is what they use at

Dignitas, so it would essentially be a hipster version of the same experience.

How hard is Nembutal to obtain? Google it and, somewhere among all the dodgy-looking online pharmacies, you'll find a man called Jorge Hernandez warning you about charlatans who exploit desperate people for a quick buck. Jorge makes weekly Nembutal-sourcing trips to Mexico and seems to be motivated by a genuine desire to help tormented people live more fulfilling lives. He says his clients rarely end up taking the pill because they cherish their lives from that day forward, knowing that they can check out at a time of their choosing. But who's to say Jorge is not himself a charlatan, distinguishable from the others only by his superior sales patter? With so much at stake, you can't afford to get it wrong.

There are some entertaining characters on the suicide scene, and many crusaders who believe euthanasia should be a human right; you need to be of sound mind, however, which doesn't seem fair to me. Why should mad people like me, who often suffer terribly, be denied their rights by the suicide industry? I could see why it was important to have searching conversations with professionals (not Jorge via email, though I'm sure he'd be up for it), an audit of your life to see if there was any compelling reason for carrying on that you may not have thought of. And someone should certainly make you aware of the impact your actions will have on your family. But if madness is making your life unbearable, why should you be forced to endure it?

In a civilised society there would be suicide hotels in every community. There, in nice, bright rooms and surrounded by your loved ones, you would find peace. The founder of Dignitas, Ludwig Minelli, has spent years campaigning for the rules prohibiting the disabled and mentally ill from seeking euthanasia to be relaxed. His critics have argued that this amounts to eugenics by the back door, but he's become something of a hero to us mental incompetents. And the more I researched HD and what it was about to do to me, the more convinced I became that yes, I wanted to end my life – it was just a question of how and when.

My next stop, then, was Dr Philip Nitschke and Dr Fiona Stewart's *Peaceful Pill Handbook*, which I initially found very encouraging – who knew there were so many lethal pills, gases and tinctures? On closer examination, though, it soon became apparent that hardly any of these goodies were readily available in the UK. British people need to be quite creative in their suicides, with no guns or pills to hand. The plastic bag method was highly recommended, and seemed surer (and tidier) than jumping off a cliff. I thought about using a gas oven like Sylvia Plath, but the advent of auto-ignition meant that it would probably just have baked my head. How undignified!

I saw Dr Nitschke's Deliverance Machine at the Science Museum when I went there with the kids. I really liked the aesthetic: a J. G. Ballardesque contraption that looked like it had been beamed in from some dystopian/utopian (I wasn't sure which) future world. An old-fashioned computer monitor was hooked up to a syringe in a brief-case. The words 'If you press this button, you will receive a lethal injection and die in fifteen seconds – do you wish to proceed?' were brief and to the point. Dr Nitschke promised oblivion or your money back, which sounded like a great deal to me at the time. That very machine had helped four Australians end their lives when it was legal for about ten minutes over there. I wanted to put one on my Christmas list.

My assumption throughout all these deliberations was that I wouldn't actually be committing suicide until my symptoms had got a lot worse; I owed it to my chil-dren to keep going until then. But my mind kept drifting to scenes of peaceful self-deliverance. I'd see myself jumping from the jetty at the women's pond on Hamp-stead Heath, diving down down down like an otter and never resurfacing. Would anyone miss me? Of course they would. But the children would be better off in the long run. I couldn't bear the thought of them having to find excuses for not coming to see me when I ended up in a more commodious version of Red Oaks.

It took me a while, but I scrabbled my way up and out of depression. The atmosphere at home improved and the light bulbs seemed to last longer. I started opening the curtains and shutters every morning instead of every few weeks; for the first time in years I felt front-facing, enjoy-ing the view of the street and not minding if passers-by peered in at me. Props to Dr Ed Wild, my collaborator, for picking me up off the proverbial floor during our memorable first appointment at the HD clinic in the National Hospital for Neurology and Neurosurgery, and edging me out of denial with warmth and tact. We talked for about an hour and he asked a lot of personal questions, but somehow they didn't feel intrusive. I related the kitchen-sink drama unfolding at home with no omissions and he listened sympathetically.

I was both relieved *and* upset to discover that my unhinged behaviour was actually quite normal for an HD person. This time I couldn't be cross with Susan, or even myself. Ed told me that the psychological and behavioural symptoms of HD could be addressed by a combination of drugs and lifestyle shifts, making me feel positive about my outlook for the first time in years. To the antidepressants and mood stabilisers I'd been prescribed by the psychiatrist (who hadn't attributed the depression to HD), he added antipsychotics to douse the flames of anger. He also lobbied my GP to prescribe a range of pills for my insomnia, including zopiclone. This all proved to be a lot more effective than mindfulness.

And there were other things I could do to help myself. Simplifying my life as Ed had advised, I reduced my work commitments and explained to my editors that I couldn't work to deadlines or get to meetings on time. I thought that this would mean the end of my journalistic career, but I was pleasantly surprised by their response.

One small but significant lifestyle shift was to get rid of my signature bob. I had my hair cut short, which felt liberating. No longer a slave to my straighteners, I had time to spend doing the things I enjoyed, like singing in a folk choir. I am a terrible singer, but I liked the way it felt to sing with one voice and be part of a collective that was greater than the sum of its parts. I stood at the back and lip synced to 'She Moves Through the Fair' and 'Blow the Winds'. Anna was as scornful of this development as John was enthusiastic. Touchingly, he came to all our concerts and even sat through the Morris dancing without fidgeting, which is hard to do at any age. He was the youngest person there by a big margin and easily the best dressed, in high-street skinny jeans that were in pleasing contrast to all the earnest hand-knitted jumpers.

If I'd had a 'peaceful pill' in a locked box in the loft, would I have taken it when I was at my lowest? I'm sure the promise of deliverance would have been alluring. The suicide rate for HD sufferers is higher than for any other neurodegenerative illness, and suicidal thoughts are most likely to occur within a few months of the initial diagnosis.

This corresponds with my experience. Since I climbed out of my depression there has been a period of relative stability where I've found I can be philosophical about my limitations and even welcome the lessons they can teach me. The future suddenly looks bearable, if not exactly bright. I've stopped picturing my glamorous funeral with a coach and four pulling my coffin up the high street because I've realised it was an attempt to transfer control of the narrative from HD to me. As well as being discourteous to the children, killing myself would have looked like hubris – a PR stunt, an attempt at self-promotion. Living with HD will be a huge challenge but I am curious about how the story will unfold.

6

Family

I have a happy recurring dream that injects sadness into my mornings because, for a millisecond after I wake up, the set-up I have dreamed about feels real. In the dream, Susan and Murph have died but me and Dan and some of our creative friends have decided to live in my old family home in Brighton. My *Feminist Times* colleague is one of them, and a young musician whose work I admire, and the old university friend who contacted me via my blog because he was concerned about me. They're all happy to move down from London to live in Brighton with me. There's no mortgage so they can live with me rent-free.

We soon set up quite an interesting scene, and I am relieved to escape the loneliness of my fractured nuclear family in favour of a radical collective – it feels like the commune in Cornwall one of my friends ran away to. The others are all happy for me to have the best room, Susan and Murph's, with its view of the garden and Brighton beyond. The room is bathed in sunlight and I feel both completely myself and completely at home, with people who share my sense of humour and appreciate me. It's a fresh start, like people in soap operas always get. What has happened to the children? They aren't in this picture. Perhaps they're living with Tom. When I wake up, I am angry with him in his absence. In the dream, justice had been done. This wasn't what happened in real life, as we will discover.

Two months after Murph died I was waiting for John to come out of a ballet class when I found out by email that Dan and I had been disinherited. Murph had left his mortgage-free house to Lottie. I'd known that he'd changed his will two years after meeting her, but it was still a shock to see it in black and white. Along with all the other emotions, there was a pit-of-the-stomach fear about the future. It meant I would be dependent on Tom for the rest of my life, wherever the tide took our relationship, and that wasn't a nice feeling.

There were some strange things in the will. A pub friend who hadn't visited Murph at Red Oaks because he'd found it 'too upsetting' was given more money than Anna, and there was nothing for John. In his final days, Murph had seemed very worried about me and kept asking weird questions about how much Tom earned – assuming we would stay together, of course. It was now clear why he'd been feeling so anxious.

Scary letters from Lottie's lawyer made me lose sleep. Apparently, there wasn't enough left in the estate to pay her legacy. Murph had lent us some of the money to buy our house in Kentish Town, so we would need to sell it and pay Lottie back out of the proceeds. We considered challenging the will but our lawyer said there were no grounds for doing so, as Murph hadn't given me any money for years. It all felt very unfair. I had HD with care costs that were certain to escalate – plus, of course, there was a chance the children might have it too.

After more than a year of worrying and feeling precarious, the lawyers finally found a way for Lottie to get her money and us to keep the house. It was a huge relief, but the whole experience had been bruising and draining. Tom said that instead of thinking about what I didn't have, I should concentrate on what I did; there was something tyrannical about his positivity that I'd started to resent rather than welcome. His ban on complaining wasn't lifted as my life got worse.

Tom's family is multiplying while mine is diminishing. Apart from Dan, there are no Ravens on my father's side left in the UK. Two of my uncles died young and the other one moved to Australia in his twenties, so I grew up knowing nothing about him. The decision to give Anna and John the Sheahan name was made by tossing a coin, but now I feel like I should have contested it; I often find myself wishing they were Ravens, which is a better name and easier to spell when you are talking to the bank. It is also cooler, clearly. Anna is planning to redress the balance by getting a tattoo of a raven on her shoulder.

Ravens are an endangered species. Tom's huge family have been very supportive towards me but they have a different way of life and aren't blood. The Raven way of life has no religious motivation for being kind. Our family culture is hard to encapsulate: it is sedentary, with endless talking and very little doing. Our group identity was forged in a crucible of cryptic catchphrases and kitchen-table conversations about politics and popular culture. We drink.

The Sheahans are sober but not sombre: they listen to classical music and engage in wholesome middle-class pastimes throughout the year. Cakes are baked and prize-winning vegetables nurtured. Granny belongs to a book group and I enjoy talking to her about the novels she's read but, in spite of some overlapping tastes, it rarely feels like we really 'get' each other. The whole family are evangelical about the benefits of fresh air and low-level discomfort. Striding forth in Berghaus shorts and brandishing Ordnance Survey maps, they relish rough terrain and choppy seas. They are anti-consumerist and can be judgemental of those of us who stray into designer clothes shops. They feel morally superior to the 'morons' chasing brands, which I don't – I often find myself siding with the teenagers in debates about Westfield and mobile phones (in fact, I often sit with them at family dinners as a show of solidarity).

They are all quite small and I am quite tall so I feel like Alice in Wonderland when I go to their second home, a cottage in Dorset where all the furniture was bought second hand forty years ago. I bang my head on the low beams and can't get out of the armchair because the seat has sunk to the floor after so many years of service. The springs stick out of the sofa. There is no central heating. The living-room carpet is a doormat. I once fell through a garden chair that must have been bought in the 70s. It's impossible to clean because the vacuum cleaner is a 60s model that actually spits out dust (we saw the same one in the Museum of Childhood). I stopped going there because it's such a long way from here, and because there are more of us than can be comfortably accommodated. I was committed to my view of the place, whatever the consequences. But I didn't like Tom and the children going without me and leaving me on my own.

I have often entertained people with stories about the infelicities of the cottage, but I was missing the point: Tom spent all his childhood summers there and the atmosphere is warm and welcoming. You can feel the love when you walk in. And my children used to love it there – no one had to worry about spilling Ribena on the carpet because there wasn't one. John carried on loving it when teenage Anna grew less keen. Tom blamed me for her change of heart, as her moaning about the lack of TV, heating and phone reception sounded uncannily like my own routine.

It couldn't have been more different from my father's second home in Florida. Where the Sheahans' cottage was a product of middle-class/Catholic guilt about the whole idea of even having a second home, Murph's condo reflected his justifiable working-class pride at having 'made it' when he sold the business he had built up. The house was in a clean, characterless gated community on Longboat Key. It had a massive TV and a La-Z-Boy for him to lounge in while he was watching CNN. Beyond the back yard there was a golf course; he would sit on his terrace with a gin and tonic and wave at the seniors as they went by in their golf buggies, admiring the pelicans on the artificial lake. We all hated it there but Murph didn't care, and I respected him for that. More than anything, he wanted to be safe and comfortable. It was like a footballer's house, with a black Thunderbird in the drive that Lottie used to roar around in. She hated the house too. It was one of the few things we all agreed on.

Murph had spent his childhood squashed into a two-up two-down in Plymouth with three brothers (there was an oft-revisited gag about them all having to share the same bowl of porridge), so it was thoroughly understandable that he had no appetite for austerity in his later years. I grew up knowing nothing about his family history; I was too self-absorbed to think about it, and that suited him. He wanted to efface HD from the record, and would have succeeded if he hadn't got ill himself. When he became symptomatic we all started asking questions, but he remained evasive. His brothers were never referred to.

His father did visit us a couple of times when I was very young, but the only thing I can remember about him now is that he brought me and Dan dates instead of sweets. My mother's family were part of our lives, but we never seemed to have much in common with them – her brother was a maths prodigy and chess champion who had married a devout Christian. Susan's mother was given to darkly muttering, after a few drinks, 'I have secrets I will take to my grave', to which Susan would invariably reply, 'If you mean Mick's not my father, I've always known.' I think she must have intuited this because her brother – who *was* Mick's – had always been favoured throughout their childhood. After Susan's death, her mother was more forthcoming, but not much: she still wouldn't tell us the real father's name, but we did learn that he had been rich. And married.

As for Murph, I finally plucked up the courage to press him on the ellipses in his backstory on one of our trips to Florida, after Susan's death but before his diagnosis. We were drinking weak daiquiris in a posh but charmless bar on St Armands Key. His face clouded over when I asked about his mother but he eventually disclosed that her name had been Ida, and she'd been 'schizophrenic' (whether or not he knew this to be a misdiagnosis at the time, I'll never know). As hard as that was to hear, it at least explained why he'd never talked nostalgically about his childhood. I wondered if repression had made his traumatic memories inaccessible to him. Viewed from a certain angle, his whole personality might have been a construct that was created as a defence – an affable false self that never wanted to argue and was always in a good mood. He rarely read novels or watched films because he was interested in facts, not feelings.

He seemed less reserved in his later years, and would probably have told me anything if his medication hadn't robbed him of the power of speech. I managed to glean a little more about Ida from him, but it took my Australian uncle Colin to fill in the missing pieces. Colin is a retired linoleum salesman who's more candid than Murph ever was, although his wife says he never talked about his childhood either until recently. He is a larger-than-life character with a loud voice and a persuasive manner who couldn't be more different from my dad; where Murph was enigmatic, he is straightforward. Opinion is divided on whether there is a physical resemblance (I think the jawline is similar).

Colin got in touch with me because he wanted to know everything about his family. He had spent the last couple of years on ancestry.com, tracing the line back and firing off letters to family friends. These efforts had yielded a picture of his and Murph's grandmother (who, I was pleased to discover, looked like an olden-days lesbian with short hair and broad shoulders) beside her elegant, consumptive-looking sister, who died young. But there was no picture of Ida.

By chance I came across Peter Congdon's *A Bomb in a Basket*, a memoir that recounts the six years of the Second World War as seen through the eyes of a child growing up in Plymouth. I just thought it would be good background reading to give me a flavour of life in Murph's home town, so I was surprised and delighted to discover that Peter had actually been a good friend of the Ravens, who feature prominently in the book. This description of Ida, from the chapter 'Plymouth on the Front Line', made me cry:

Reg had married Ida in the early 30s. She was a strange woman with a deep voice, and rumour had it she had been a nurse. Although apparently educated and articulate, Ida presented as a shabbily dressed lady who was often to be seen smoking cigarettes. Her standards of hygiene, cleanliness and housework were not of the highest quality and much of the responsibility for running the home was left to Reg, who was often seen shopping for the family. At the time, little did we know that Ida was suffering from a serious mental illness that was to worsen over the years.

According to Colin, she hardly ever left the house. I can picture her on a battered divan ('in her misery', in Colin's phrase) with no pharmaceutical props, chain-smoking while family life went on around her. The radio was always on (Ida liked radio dramas) and Peter Congdon said it was like Liberty Hall compared to his house: in the boys' bedroom they would take turns to jump onto the bed from the top of the wardrobe.

Colin said Ida was embarrassing. She did weird things that were well intentioned, like making a lurid pink blancmange 'birthday cake' for Murph's birthday and decorating it with large household candles (everyone who ate it was sick). When she picked them up from school they were always painfully conscious of her dirty dress and wraithlike appearance, and she used to eat porridge straight out of the packet. But they never doubted how much she loved them.

The most upsetting thing about all this in retrospect is that no one ever realised Ida had HD, because it just wasn't widely known about then – the best anyone could do was fall back on the same 'schizophrenia' diagnosis Murph had tried to palm me off with in Florida. As a result, she ended up spending two long stretches at Moorhaven Asylum in Ivybridge, near Plymouth. It looked like a grand country house with lots of outbuildings, beautiful views across the moor, a farm and its own railway station. But it was still a madhouse.

What was life like for Ida there? Was her treatment plan appropriate? I pictured Nurse Ratched from *One Flew Over the Cuckoo's Nest* and a daily diet of chemical coshes – not to mention ECT, which was at the height of its popularity in the 40s. Looking for reassurance, I did some research and came across a social history project called 'Memories of Moorhaven'. Some people had happy memories of the place but suicide was apparently so common that everyone got quite blasé about it. They were always scraping people off the railway tracks.

Had Ida gone there voluntarily? Colin doesn't know. All he remembers about visiting her there is the smell of disinfectant and the fact that she seemed quite calm, but Murph remembered it as 'grim'. Was she longing for their visits?

Back home in Townsend Avenue, the Raven house was managing to survive the blitz but life still felt precarious. Murph's playgrounds were bombed-out buildings and he used to do his homework sitting on the shelter in the yard, looking insouciant. Perhaps it was even for the best that Ida had been sent to the countryside, away from the danger – people with HD like things to be predictable, and stress can exacerbate the symptoms. Murph was himself briefly evacuated to Cambourne roughly halfway through the war, and we still have a letter he sent to his father while he was away. His handwriting is more legible than my son's; I'm not sure how old he was. He says he's ahead of Colin at school but Colin is catching up, and he signs off with forty-two kisses.

The more I found out about Murph's childhood, the sorrier I felt for him. He must have looked neglected, and I couldn't bear to think of him being bullied by his classmates for his dishevelment. But many of these fears were allayed when I finally found out a bit more about Reg, his amazing father.

On one of Colin's rare visits to the UK, a few months before Murph died, we visited Red Oaks and the two elder Ravens were in the mood to reminisce, fleshing Reg out for me. By all accounts he was a diamond who'd been dealt a bad hand but made the best of it. A guard on the Great Western Railway, he loved his job but had to walk for miles to get to work, and often fell asleep when he got there. I'm not surprised – upon returning home in the evening he would cook, clean, scrub the front steps and do whatever else it took to look after Ida and the four boys. This gender role reversal probably raised some eyebrows in the neighbourhood but I'm lost in admiration for him. He was often to be seen walking up the hill with a sack of potatoes on his back, and his Cornish pasties were legendary. Without this committed and tolerant optimist at the helm of the family, Murph's story could have been very different.

Why weren't Reg and his dates a bigger part of my life when I was growing up? Had Murph fallen out with him, or was their apparent estrangement just standard behaviour for stoical working-class men of their respective generations? Either way, I'm sorry to have missed out on him – as I write, there's a picture of him in his GWR uniform on my desk.

Moorhaven Asylum has been turned into a quirky, upscale housing development called Moorhaven Village. I visited it to see whether Ida's ghost was stalking the remodelled bedrooms. It was pouring with rain and the kids were moaning (we were en route to a festival); they stayed in the car as I walked glumly about, trying to picture Ida doing exercises on the lawn like the inmates in the pictures I'd found. I still hadn't managed to find a picture of Ida herself, and this was beginning to be a source of real sadness for me. If my HD test had been negative I might have gone to my grave without ever thinking about her, but genetic conditions create a chain of association. I felt a connection to her now, so it was dispiriting to think that I might never see her face.

I respect the Sheahans more than I used to. I came around to them just as Tom was going off me, which was inconvenient for everyone. Apart from being kind, they are ethical and outward-facing. Tom's sister, Frances, is a funny and warm human rights lawyer and they all have a global perspective. There are so many of them, though; a gathering becomes a melee. I went on one family holiday where there were fifteen people around the table at mealtimes and six children sharing a bedroom. I was brought up in a small family where you could always hear what everyone was saying.

I think Anna and John got the best bits of the Sheahan and Raven cultures without any of the Sheahan scruples or Raven spiritual laziness. Anna is practical and political, so I was surprised when she said she wanted to join the army cadets and shocked when she stuck at it for a year, progressing through the ranks until she became a lance corporal in 2018. How did she deal with being told what to do? It would have been inconceivable for me to defer to any authority figure when I was thirteen. If they'd shouted at me, I would have shouted back or sniggered disdainfully at the very least. But Anna kept on taking herself off to the barracks twice a week and, in spite of myself, I was proud to see the care with which she ironed her uniform. The whole thing seemed genuinely character-building, and the way she described the pleasure of marching in time with 400 people made it sound like the same sense of collective purpose I experience on demos: a riposte to individualism.

John is charming, funny and a self-confessed show-off, with morbid preoccupations that I'm not sure whether to be alarmed by. The people who have looked after him over the years have enjoyed being part of his imaginative world and marvelling at his core strength when he demonstrates his acrobatic dance moves. I'm not sure what to attribute his fascination with death and the end of the world to, but Anna suspects him of putting it on to impress me. It's certainly true that, as a former goth, I am pale with pride when he demonstrates the 'hanging man' pose on the makeshift trapeze Tom set up for him in our garden.

Dan has been a frequent visitor to our house in Kentish Town, and we really look forward to seeing him. The children like him because he never does any exercise (despite living in a flat by the sea) and is a computer game connoisseur. I appreciate him more than I used to and no longer talk over him, literally or metaphorically. I feel guilty about being a terrible sister for all those years; he doesn't want me to, though. We became friends in middle age, which was a pleasure neither of us had expected. I've alienated so many people, some irretrievably, that Dan's forgiveness has had a big impact on me, making me feel like redemption is possible. My house feels like our old childhood home in Brighton when he's here.

I'm trying to remember how Anna and John came to know about HD. There was no shroud of secrecy or 'not in front of the children' when they were younger. As I've said, I remember the day when Murph's friend told me about his diagnosis, but I don't think Anna and John would be able to pinpoint it so precisely. I wanted our approach to be honest without over-sharing, which I have a tendency to do. I didn't want to burden them with too much hard-to-process information at the wrong time or in an age-inappropriate way. On the other hand, as Susan's daughter, I wanted to tell the truth. My behaviour must have seemed hard to account for so I figured it might actually come as a relief to them to find out about the HD, and I think it did. There was no big reveal but rather a controlled release of information, conveyed in digestible portions over time. We answered questions as they came up. Of course, it was easier to tell them about my illness than the fact that they were both at risk of developing it too.

I sometimes wonder if John's obsession with death has anything to do with the fact that he was made aware of my mortality and his own at such a young age. For our family, the end of days is always close at hand. 'We are all going to die, Mum. It's either a meteor hitting the planet or the bees dying, or droughts or plastic pollution or sea levels rising.' He is cross with the adults for destroying the planet and feels impotent because there's nothing he can do that will influence what happens. He might feel the same about the looming threat of HD and be cross with me without being able to express it. Anna wants to be tested for the gene when she is old enough. I have reassured them both that, by that time, drugs will be available that treat the illness and not just the symptoms. Is this true, though? The advances in gene science Ed spoke about when I saw him at the clinic sounded promising, but he couldn't commit to a timescale.

As the illness progressed, they both helped me. Anna drew on the first aid she'd learned at cadets to look after me when I burned myself. She also pulled a splinter out of my foot with a pin, very adeptly. When I dropped a tumbler in the basin upstairs, John removed the tiny bits of glass from the plughole with tweezers and even complimented me on my comparative cool-headedness ('I'm proud of you, Mum – you dealt with it very well'). He is always thinking of me and I sometimes worry that he prioritises my happiness over his own. The birthday teas he throws for me are beautiful, with menus and proper china; I am allowed to play my playlist and there is always a Cirque de Soleil-inspired show. The way he treats me, it feels like my birthday every day.

Friends have asked me if Susan was aware of the looming threat of HD before she died. I don't think she was – Murph's 'don't ask, don't tell' policy about his childhood was surprisingly effective. Sometimes I'm glad she died without knowing what was to come, but she was practical, committed and good in a crisis. If she'd been alive, I've no doubt she would have looked after Murph throughout his illness.

I can see her tending to him thoughtfully, and never getting bored or frustrated by the repetitive strain of caring for someone with HD. It would have been a matter of pride to her not to outsource his care. When I became symptomatic, she could have stepped into Tom's role with more time than he ever had to support me in the years when I was declining and struggling with everyday tasks. There is plenty of room at my house so she could have stayed with me for long stretches, and the carers who have bored and irritated me could have been stood down. She was a brilliant cook and a stabilising presence, and I think she would have loved her grandchildren.

They often ask about her. The balance of Ravens to Sheahans in their lives has changed, with the Sheahan way of doing things now predominant. Thank goodness for Dan, the Last Great Raven. He may not be very practical but he knows a hawk from a handsaw, and more than makes up for the fact that he can't cook by being such a fun guest. When he visits, I feel I can be myself.

In late 2016, Colin called with some good news: he'd finally found a picture of Ida. It was taken before she became symptomatic so she's in her nurse's uniform, looking healthy and happy. I would have put her picture next to Reg's on my desk whatever it had turned out to look like, but I'm so glad it turned out to look like that. Colin said he took it to a beach near where he lives in Sydney, to say goodbye to her. His caption: 'Ida Raven – Lost and Found'.

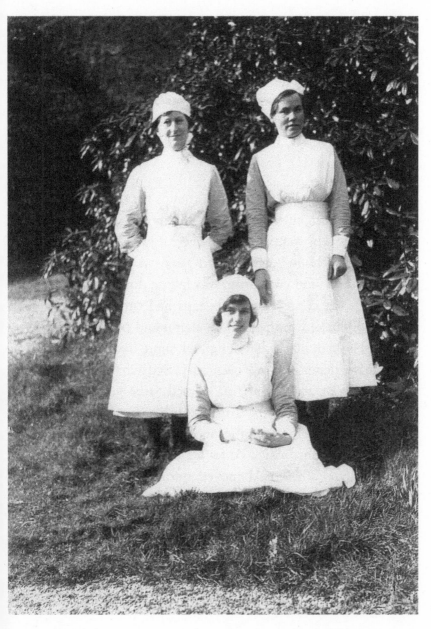

My grandmother Ida (centre), in the era when she was caring for other people

7

Anxiety

Tom and I had agreed to stay friends for the sake of the children, which meant family dinners twice a week at the house in Kentish Town where I now lived without him. The house, whose renovation we had embarked upon as a joint enterprise, was falling down around my ears – the contentious Vola taps had run dry and the hand-blocked wallpaper was damp and peeling. Nothing worked; our grand design felt more like a prison.

My friends had all been surprised when we finally split up in 2018. 'But you seemed to be getting on so well,' they'd said, one after the other. In the past year there had been a lot of toing and froing with different configurations, which I'd found unsettling and anxiety-inducing. When he'd moved onto that houseboat, I hadn't really expected him to return. But return he had, and together we'd implemented the model of collaborative co-parenting and mutual support we'd agreed on in our last session of marriage therapy, separated but under the same roof. I'd thought that it had been working for everyone, so when Tom declared that he wasn't happy I was devastated. He said he couldn't move on while we were in the same house, which was obviously true.

John now lives with Tom in a flat over the road, although he comes back to me every Friday and for one weekend a month. Tom and I generally spend that weekend doing stuff together with the children, which seemed like a good idea in theory. One Sunday during the holidays, when Anna was away, we went to IKEA to buy beds for Tom and John's new flat. There were pregnant women around every bend, and all the happy families were engaged in domestic simulations in those weird rooms where they stage visions of Nordic harmony. What a terrible idea. How could he expect me to be cheerful? We were furnishing his new life!

I shouldn't have said what I was thinking but I did, and instantly regretted it as John looked stricken. There was a long queue at the till and I was hungry so I went with him to look for food. We queued for half an hour at a food station by the entrance that was selling lurid hot dogs and super-sweet fake marzipan pastries with a weird taste and texture called 'Memorable Moments with Laughter and Pastries'. This was inarguably a memorable moment. John felt sick after a couple of bites so I took him outside. He said, 'I'm allergic to that thing.'

In the van on the way back to Kentish Town, my anxiety levels began to rise at the prospect of returning with Anna to the house that was too big for just the two of us. It was hard to feel enthusiastic about the housewarming tea with our mutual friends and their children that Tom would be hosting on his new roof terrace beforehand.

My forty-ninth birthday party was an old-school affair with cocktails, drugs and arguments about playlists. Tom bought me a Bluetooth speaker that I found tricky to operate. Before I could work it out, Anna and John had set up camp on it and were, as usual, refusing to let me play my esoteric 90s bleepcore and experimental folk.

After everyone had gone, Tom helped me find the Valium I had been buying off the internet and the pills I took for my various HD symptoms, then asked if I needed help undressing. In the bathroom upstairs he encouraged me to clean my teeth and put the brush back on its charger in the same voice he would have used with Anna or John. Was this patronising or kind? He washed the mouthguard that stopped me grinding my teeth, which was a must if I'd taken coke. I felt like a child rather than a wife – cared for but no longer longed for.

This shift in the status of our relationship was hard to bear. My bedroom was an echo chamber of memories from our scented candle/fairy lights on the mirror/Agent Provocateur era, when I was still alive. HD had nullified my sexuality; I was still capable of intimacy, though. I could have reconciled myself to losing one of those essential aspects of humanity but not both. The private jokes, long spooling conversations that never went anywhere and other affirming aspects of my relationship with Tom had all gone, and no one ever hugged or even touched me apart from John (Anna hates being hugged, even by relatives).

The help Tom gave me on my birthday night was appreciated, but it left me unconsoled. Weirdly, I think it was as sad for him as it was for me. When he asked, 'Is there anything else you need before I go?', I silently screamed, 'Yes!' but ended up saying, 'No thanks, I'm fine. That was a great party. I'm pleased you were there.' He said he would come back in the morning to help me clear up and then, in the blink of an eye, he was gone.

I had a restless and tormented night. I knew I was cross with him but it took me a while to work out why: he'd talked to me as if I were more disabled than I was. It was infantilising, and perhaps even subtly controlling. But it had always been important for him to feel like he was in charge of us all.

I had lost my self-esteem and my identity was imperilled. I didn't know who I was any more, and I was battling with the pain of rejection every day. Everyone agreed that I should take my wedding pictures down from the mantelpiece and get rid of the dress, which was still in my wardrobe – how could I move on without doing that? – but the physical act of putting them in either storage or the rubbish would have been so charged with unwelcome symbolism that I just couldn't face it.

People kept asking me if I was going to start 'dating', and this really annoyed me. I couldn't meet anyone because I never left the house! Tinder would have been impossible and scary, and HD had taken my smile. I needed to be realistic about my prospects: I was undateable, and feeling unlovable. Who would want a completely companionate arrangement, where sex was off the agenda, with a person suffering from a degenerative brain disease? I couldn't talk on the phone, or walk down the street without falling over and hurting myself, or make a sandwich, or cut my own nails, or find my way anywhere, or manage my finances, or get anywhere on time, or read, or look after my children, or eat anything without spilling it all over me.

I was surprised by how many of the people at the support group had committed spouses who were present and looking after them; their small acts of tenderness were evidence of intimacy continuing against the odds. Some of these couples were struggling financially and trying to navigate a hostile benefit environment for people with disabilities. I would have felt guilty if Tom had given up work to look after me – and it would have been a disaster, because we'd have lost the house and everything else. But I wouldn't have felt as anxious, as there was no substitutable stranger who could reassure me the way he always had. I needed to learn self-sufficiency halfway through this degenerative illness, which seemed very unfair.

HD traps me in banality, as boring things take five times longer than they used to and interesting things are no longer accessible. I gave up going to my choir because I couldn't learn the words or remember the tunes; I missed the friends I'd made there, who had shared my politics. Apathy made it hard for me to get out of bed, and when

I did finally make it I'd get tangled up in my clothes or put them on the wrong way around. Social services assessed me at some point and agreed that I needed help with many everyday tasks, even though I looked okay.

Carers were a mixed blessing at first. It took a while for us to find people who both understood HD and empathised with me. My first agency carer freely admitted that she hated her job, and seemed to be going through some sort of mid-life crisis. She talked and talked about her other clients, her alcoholic son and her colourful life back home in South Africa before she came to the UK. Her husband had killed someone in a bar brawl. How could my anecdotes compete with that? Our relationship was claustrophobic; I did have a laugh with her, though.

I wanted the people 'working with me' to enjoy hanging out with me, then worried when my relationships with them lost their boundaries. But that's not always a bad thing, and some carers have stayed the distance to become supportive friends. Ade has a vintage stall on Portobello Road, selling beautiful clothes she sources from charity shops; when the shit hit the fan and I was anxious about everything every day, she'd distract me by talking to me about clothes. She's also a trained counsellor who has worked with survivors of the Grenfell Tower fire. Because I had a lot of respect for her, I found it difficult to ask her to cook or clean or do anything else she might not enjoy doing. I sometimes wished she were more of a carer and less of a friend, so I wouldn't feel so guilty about asking her to do things for me.

Recognising that I was also going to need support outside office hours, Tom paid an agency to find me a housemate who could help with meals and the children in the evenings. He thought he was doing his duty by hiring Lucy, but having someone paid to be here who I didn't have much in common with was actually worse than being on my own. It certainly wasn't like having a husband. I was no longer welcome on family holidays because Tom says everyone would have a miserable time if I came: 'It's not fair on them. You won't be on your own, you'll have your carers.' But not my children. He has said a lot of cruel things that I find it difficult to forgive or forget ('You being lonely is not my responsibility'). I don't think he realises the impact they've had on me.

The early days of the post-Tom era were characterised by a strange combination of realism and anxiety: I'd accepted that I was ill but felt fearful about the future. And the existential dread that came with the end of denial about the seriousness of my condition was inevitably compounded when I also had to stop denying that Tom didn't want me any more. He dealt with most of the logistics of the separation so I wouldn't have to get stressed, but that just meant there wasn't anything to distract me from my situation. I couldn't read anything longer than a blog post and was bored out of my mind most of the time, which was hard to convey to my carers.

The therapist who'd wept at me was replaced by someone with experience of people with long-term health conditions, specifically neurological illnesses and strokes. Jason, who had been recommended by one of my carers, was a clinical psychologist rather than a counsellor, and his prices reflected his expertise – I could only afford to see him once a fortnight. Getting there was a bit of a mission as he worked near Liverpool Street Station, which is quite a distance from Kentish Town. I was late for our first session because the Uber didn't drop me in the right place; Jason retrieved me from the street, where I was wandering around and about to get very lost. I was in a terrible state, too anxious to relate the circumstances that had brought me to him.

I stopped compulsively texting Tom but had no one else to turn to for reassurance apart from Anna – and it didn't seem fair to assign her the role of Reassurer-in-Chief at such a young age. Tom's flat over the road might as well have been a million miles away. I wished there had been a ritual or way of saying goodbye that wasn't such a sudden rupture, and lobbied for this before realising that it was a big ask. A few weeks before he left he'd come back from one of his trips without his wedding ring, and it had been a complete shock.

While googling HD and anxiety I came across a website by a specialist whose stated aim was to educate and empower doctors who don't realise that many of the symptoms can be effectively managed by drugs. 'Huntington's MD' said that general anxiety was a common feature of HD but that mood stabilisers could be an effective treatment, as could antidepressants teamed with antipsychotics. Mirtazapine was recommended; Ed had already prescribed that but I was still anxious. For more severe cases, Huntington's MD said that benzodiazepine could be useful. I had already failed to persuade my GP to prescribe me that so I looked for it online. It was only a couple of clicks away and was delivered within a couple of days.

I took 10mg a night and have never slept better. I'd have a fuzzy head the next day, which made it hard to think, but that was a price I was willing to pay for peace of mind and spirit. I would have carried on taking it if Ed hadn't told me off ('I'm not telling you off') – weirdly, this medical professional counselled against buying drugs online! I was so cross with him for not empathising with my predicament that I started telling *him* off: my freedom of movement had been curtailed by anxiety, what else was I meant to do? If he'd suggested mindfulness, as Jason had on what proved to be our last session, I would have left the room.

He said it would be a bad idea to continue with the Valium because I would have to keep on increasing the dose – addiction would be inevitable, and the withdrawal sounded pretty awful (one of the withdrawal symptoms was anxiety!). But in the same consultation he told me some exciting news, dispensing hope and a cautiously presented promise of deliverance that couldn't have been better timed. I'd noticed that the mood at the HD clinic had lifted from downbeat to optimistic and I wasn't sure why. After years of false starts and blind alleys and watching their patients decline and die with no hope of a cure, Ed and his colleagues had made an era-defining breakthrough in gene therapy and were trialling a gene silencing drug.

The science was hard to grasp. Their hope for the drug was that it would slow the progression of the disease and possibly even reverse it, as it had in some HD mice used in the early trials. When it was eventually tested on humans, the results were so remarkable that they soon became headline news all over the world. I was carried along on a wave of excitement. Friends kept emailing me to see if I'd seen the papers. Some of them sounded cautious, hoping that it wasn't fake news – I was pleased to reassure them that, for once, the hype was justified.

The next step would be to see if the drug worked on a larger cohort. I wasn't sure how many people they would be recruiting for this or when the trial would start, but I knew I wanted to be part of it. Even if I turned out to be one of the people who got the placebo, it would give me a sense of purpose – and I needed something meaningful to do instead of just 'looming', as Anna calls it. Ed said I would be a good candidate as I still had reasonably good motor control and balance, and my cognitive impairments weren't severe. My medication would have to be stable for three months before the trial commenced, though – another good reason to get off the Valium, and presumably cocaine would be off limits too. Nightmare!

And, well, surely everyone else who had HD (and could still understand the news) would be trying to get on the trial too? Knowing about it while also understanding that it would be unethical for Ed to shoe-horn me onto it was difficult. It sounded like a big commitment, as there would be monthly injections in the spine and lots of appointments to go to. I would need to find a 'trial buddy' to support me. Clearly this couldn't be Tom. Who could I ask?

Meanwhile I was back to my old anxious self, only now I was anxious about not getting on the trial. I didn't dare read any of Ed's articles on HDBuzz about gene silencing. Without the Valium there was a hard-to-deal-with amplification of anxiety: what had previously been a background hum was now white noise. It was impossible to hear what anyone was saying over it, including myself. I felt it settling into my home like an uninvited guest. Although Tom had done his best to keep us on an even keel by employing a nanny and carers, there were times when I was on my own with the children and anxiety blotted them out.

Anxiety is contagious. John has been through phases of being anxious, and even Lucy, my housemate, noticed that she worried more when she started living with me. On a trip to the V&A one Sunday, we all panicked when we got to the café and realised that my purse wasn't in my bag. I must have left it on the Tube! Lucy and John were trying to get me to think it through calmly. John said, 'They have a lost property place, won't it be there?' I said that if anyone found it, they'd nick it. We called Anna to see if I'd left it at home. I had! What a relief. On the Tube back, Lucy must have checked to see if her purse and mobile were in her bag about a hundred times.

We were relying on public transport because I had already crashed the car and written it off. This happened years before my lack of coordination and inability to multitask would have stopped me from driving – thinking back, it may have been an expression of anxiety rather than a genuine loss of motor control. Tom had been away for four weeks, filming a reality show in Panama, and I wasn't coping, so I crashed into a bollard on the Holloway Road. Perhaps, subconsciously, I wanted to show him that he *couldn't* be away and uncontactable – bad things would happen if he was. So my anxiety had tried to curtail his freedom of movement too.

The children were pleased when I stopped driving because the school run had been hair-raising for years, and we're very well served by buses and Tubes in Kentish Town. I could have got to the West End in half an hour any time I wanted to – it was the wanting to that was lacking.

Anxiety governed my life, stopping me from going anywhere or doing anything. I'd even feel scared about going to the monthly HD support group, which was only/horribly a bus ride away. But I'd make myself do it, and was pleased when I did. Many of my comrades had also found their freedom of movement restricted by fear; there were touching accounts of battles with a Medusa's head of paralysing dread. At the time I looked perfectly well, with no visible disability, but my world had shrunk. I'd tried to detach myself emotionally from Tom, as everyone advised, but his presence had been a mood stabiliser and I couldn't think who else to nominate for the role. If Susan had been alive, I could have texted her.

Although the anxiety that HD sufferers typically feel is caused by physical changes in the brain, it can be exacerbated by changes to their routine or environment – so it was no surprise that I was struggling to settle down with everything constantly shifting around me. I wanted a routine but kept getting new carers and nannies and housemates before I had time to get used to the old ones, and they came at different times every week so I lost track of them. One of the nannies resigned, which I was pleased about as she wasn't a good fit for the family (Anna hid in her room whenever she was here and said she missed the 'bants' she'd had with the last nanny but one).

There is a unique quality to loneliness when you have nannies and carers who are constantly changing, and a housemate who's a stranger from an agency, that is hard to convey. The days when my kitchen table was encircled by smiling, sympathetic faces seem very far away. Dan is also anxious and has become more so since Murph died, but he still has no plans to get tested for the HD gene. When he comes to visit we chat late into the night, both seeking reassurance that neither of us is equipped to provide. I smoke cigarettes and he smokes dope. At least he lets me listen to my playlist.

I've tried to explain to John that it's normal to worry about things, but that my anxiety is a symptom of the illness. It's hard for him to tell the difference. The last time I took him to the dentist I had to get him to fill in the form that gave my consent for his treatment, which must have looked odd. The waiting room was full of angry people standing. They were all staring at us – this wasn't paranoia, they really were. I also couldn't remember his date of birth.

I went to a Salon London event about technology and feminism at the Hospital Club in Covent Garden, but bolted in the break rather than talk to anyone. I used to love that kind of thing but I've lost confidence and my sense of who I am. Walking back to the Tube station in the rain, I wondered if it might be possible to think differently about my illness. Maybe Tom had been right all along: assuming a more positive outlook might not be a betrayal of my Ravenishness but rather a pragmatic decision to choose life even in the midst of loss. It would be sensible to focus on the things I can do rather than the things I can't. Even more radically, I could take an interest in my altered state instead of constantly comparing the HD me to the old me and falling short.

People keep saying, 'You are not your illness' to inspire me to write about something else. A friend suggested pitching an idea I'd had about the sexual revolution a few years ago to the *Observer*. It's hard to explain why I wouldn't be able to write that piece now, even if they wanted it. I wish this wasn't the case and feel a terrible sense of loss about no longer being a journalist. I've been writing more truthfully in my blog but for a smaller audience – I'm proud of the writing but not the stats. This has been a difficult adjustment.

The truth is, like it or not, I *am* HD. It occupies your being, changing your personality and thinking. I honestly don't know if I ever will be able to write about anything else.

Is there anything to be learned from my experience? Does being aware of my mortality make me wiser than my friends? Probably not, but I do feel I'm at a crossroads where my skewed perspective might tell me something interesting about 'normality'. And it sounds clichéd but, after years of gruelling psychological work, I think I might finally be on the verge of an awakening; it hasn't quite happened yet but I feel like I'm on the right path at last. With fewer people looking at my work, I've been released from the burden of the perfectionism that always prevented me from properly expressing myself. My narcissism used to make me feel immortal, but I have been knocked off my pedestal and am more in touch with other people now than I have ever been. I'm also determined not to waste any more time regretting the past.

I want to be fully present for Anna and John instead of being half with them and half wrapped up in my intellectual grand designs. I was worried about John's anxiety but became less so when I accepted that it was better for him to live with Tom. I take him to his trapeze lesson every week – even though we always get lost on the way and I can't do small talk with the other parents, we do it! I stare at my phone as they talk proudly about their children, but I know I could still do that too. I have taken down my wedding pictures and put up pictures of John and some Class War posters a friend gave me in their place. I no longer feel like I am competing with my 90s self and can look at the covers of the magazine I (briefly) edited on my bathroom wall and other evidence of my media heyday without getting upset and longing for another fix of fame.

One Saturday in September, Dan visited and we went to a posh pizza restaurant with Tom and John. Tom took charge as he always did, choosing and ordering for all of us, which annoyed Dan. When Tom and John went back to their flat, Dan and I went back to mine. I ran up to my room to change into my tracksuit and slipped on the stairs on the way down (I have been falling quite often as there are many trip hazards in the house). Dan was sympathetic. I don't usually drink as much as him but we polished off a couple of bottles of Tesco's Finest Pinot Grigio and a bottle of vodka as we talked about how things had turned out. At 3 a.m. we danced – we both hate dancing – and hugged while 'You Got the Love' played on my new speaker. I was holding on to him for dear life and couldn't let go.

Talking to Dan, I felt reassured about the future. He said I should stop feeling shit about myself, detach from Tom, ditch some of my unsupportive friends and get a dog. I realised that, in a weird way, HD had brought us together.

I googled 'illness and identity' and found an essay by Peter Wilberg called 'Illness and Identity – the "Immune

Self" and its "Defences"'. In it, Wilberg offers a different way of thinking about illness:

> All illness begins with a sense of 'not feeling ourselves' – feeling different in a way we find discomforting and are ill at ease with. *Not feeling ourselves,* however, is a part of a natural process through which we can learn to *feel another self.* This is a fundamentally healthy and healing process, for by letting ourselves feel other, different selves to the one we normally identify with we quite literally come to feel more of 'ourselves'. We become more whole by feeling more of our whole self or 'soul' in all its sides and aspects.

For sufferers of HD and the people close to them, the challenge is to accept this 'other self' and not wish we were otherwise. My own other self may be less capable than the original, but it's also a lot more reasonable; I relate to people better and I'm easier to get along with. This is partly down to my medication, which hasn't changed in three years, but it's also connected to a change in my attitudes towards impairment and mortality. All of that tired old rubbish about living in the moment, taking each day as it comes, counting your blessings, etc., has turned out to be embarrassingly pertinent. I'm determined to make the most of whatever time I have left.

I may have grown up a little too late to save my relationship with Tom, but I still have my children and they still have me (for now). I feel cautiously optimistic about their futures, even if they do turn out to have the HD gene, because – thanks to Ed and his colleagues – there's every hope that the disease will be preventable or even curable by the time it becomes an issue for them.

Despite all this positivity, though, I still can't help feeling anxious about whether I'm going to get on the trial. Huntington's makes you want everything to happen right away (there is no ASAP with HD), so waiting to find out if I've been chosen feels torturous, but I know I can survive it if I find a way to be patient and foster stoicism. I will think about my predicament as an existential crisis through which it may be possible to chart a course – I want to find some meaning in my story, whether I get on the trial or not.

8

Doctors

Appointments can cut two ways: I know they're helping but often feel like they're wasting my time when I don't have much left. I keep having to answer the same questions, put by different people. They always ask about my mood using a special voice and a conspicuous abundance of eye contact. Would I tell them I was feeling suicidal with my children in the next room, or confess to feeling hopeless when I know from experience that saying this sets off alarm bells and makes Camden mental health services (who are surprisingly well funded) swing into action? They would call the next day, to direct me to support services and generally get on my case.

Appointments can be stressful as well as time consuming: I often need to prove I'm disabled because I don't always look it. I have a badge that asks passengers to give up their seats for me as they would for a pregnant woman, but Anna and John won't let me wear it. Getting a blue badge that my carers can use when they park was difficult, involving forms, a letter about my mobility from my GP and a physical assessment where they asked me to walk in a straight line; when it turned out I *was* able to do that, I had to explain that I wouldn't be able to for much longer.

Another sort of appointment involves benign, well-intentioned professionals 'working with me'. Some of them come to the house, which makes things easier, but there is a high turnover so I often see different people in the same role. I have psychiatrists, psychologists, speech therapists, occupational therapists, physios, a nutritionist, someone to monitor my swallowing, a podiatrist, someone to cut my fingernails, dentists, hygienists. Being ill can feel like a full-time job, with people assessing and reassessing constantly.

Applying for Universal Credit is complex and intimidating, in a way that would almost certainly have put me off if I hadn't really badly needed the money; I didn't have an income or any savings, so was naturally worried about both the present and the future. There will be no money to pay for my care.

Under the present system, all disability benefits have been rolled into Universal Credit. The first thing on the to-do list is to submit an online application form, which my carers helped me with as I can't really use the computer. Then you have an appointment at the job centre. On the way there I kept thinking about Ken Loach's film *I, Daniel Blake*, about a man who is declared unfit for work but dies while waiting for his claim to be processed; the 'RIP' placards carried by the demonstrators I then saw outside the actual job centre, bearing the names of claimants who'd actually died, suggested that this was no mere exaggeration for dramatic effect. I'd also read lots of reports in the *Guardian* about claimants who'd been sanctioned for arriving late to their interviews or failing to prove they'd applied for jobs.

I felt guilty about asking the state for help when there were so many people worse off than me. And it felt humiliating, which wasn't rational – I didn't mind taking money from Murph or Tom, so why not the government? The scene at the job centre was fraught, with an overbearing security guard making everyone edgy and scrappy. There were warnings everywhere about what would happen to you if you abused the staff, so I didn't. We went upstairs and were processed more quickly than I'd feared. The sick note that said I had a terminal illness without going into that much detail seemed to be enough for now.

They said I wouldn't need to keep presenting it every week or show them any evidence that I'd been looking for work, which was good. But in the week after the interview I kept getting emails saying that if I didn't log into my account *immediately* to answer a message they'd just sent, I might have to start the whole process again. My carers were never around when these emails arrived, so I was powerless to address them. What could be more anxiety-inducing?

They then sent a fifty-page form and told me it wasn't enough to have a sick note from the doctor – I needed to locate all the letters from Ed to prove when I had been diagnosed and how my illness had developed. I had, of course, lost those, so there was another delay while Ed's secretary made and sent me some copies. I just about managed to complete the form and get it sent off before the deadline, but then it was weeks before I heard anything back. I was grateful to be a middle-class white person with support and a safety net, who didn't need to rely on food banks while the authorities adjudicated my claim, but even with help the whole process had sent my anxiety levels through the roof. My lovely GP had warned me that I might be turned down because my disability was invisible but intimated that I'd probably win on appeal, as Daniel Blake had. *But he'd died before that happened!*

I always see the same GP nowadays and am happy to say that she's very well informed about HD, because many doctors aren't – the friends I've made at the HD support group have often felt let down by GPs who think there's nothing much anyone can do about HD. If those doctors were only able to approach this complex illness with some humility, they'd realise that there's actually quite a lot you can do to support patients through it. My GP has always been rooting for me and I feel confident that I can discuss anything with her. As well as keeping abreast of my symptoms and monitoring my decline (without alarming me), she knows all about my book, my marriage, my children and my money issues, and has never tried to bully me into looking on the bright side. She was as pleased with my new therapist as I was.

Stephen Grosz was more intelligent than my last therapist and also a fan of my writing, but that wasn't the only reason I felt like I'd finally found the right person. He was a psychoanalyst who'd written a book called *The Examined Life*, which I'd read and admired in healthier times. I knew I wasn't in the right place to free associate on a couch five times a week and definitely couldn't afford it – his consultation room was in Hampstead! – but he really put me at ease. I sat on a wooden chair that was more comfortable than it looked and poured my heart out to him.

Although I'd expected Stephen to be a good listener, I hadn't imagined that he'd also advise me on my life or help me work through the dilemmas that were paralysing me – but that's exactly what he did. He told me off for feeling guilty about the past and recommended seeing a couples' therapist with Tom, which seemed an excellent idea. I wanted to discuss the past, my needs in the present, what was best for the children and how things should work in the future. But how could I get Tom to go?

The couples' therapist we'd already seen (before the split) had helped us to come up with a workable plan. Leading separate lives under the same roof, where I was still supported and the children looked after, was an audacious idea that had seemed to succeed against the odds. For a few months there it really had seemed as if we'd never got on better. I was devastated when Tom said he still wasn't happy.

As well as giving me good advice, Stephen told me how I came across to him, and I was pleased to hear that the intellectual and emotional distinguishing marks that make me who I am were still intact. I left the sessions feeling less chaotic and anxious than when I'd gone in. I also felt empowered enough to enact his prescriptions for creating an intellectually and emotionally fulfilling life for myself; I had my hand on the tiller for the first time, with no one to consult about which direction I should go in, which was scary but also exciting. I was going to start with small decisions, to get the hang of them, before working up to bigger ones.

Like anyone with a long-term health condition, I spend a lot of time in waiting rooms, which means I have a lot of time to observe other patients writhing and pitching in their wheelchairs with family or carers supporting them. As much as I pity them, I'm also slightly envious because I'm always there on my own and this will remain the case when I deteriorate.

The waiting room of the HD clinic at the National Hospital is particularly hard to navigate because it's always so busy. My carer recently took me there for my yearly assessment appointment with the team from Enroll-HD, a study that aims to improve doctors' understanding of the disease by collecting clinical data and biological samples. I never look forward to this as you can tell just from their faces that you're performing worse across the board. This time I felt like I'd flunked all of the physical and cognitive tests, but ended up passing one because I could still walk (though not in a straight line any more).

Then came the inevitable questions about my mood. I had grown used to lying about this as Ed had told me you couldn't qualify for the trial if you were depressed. I thought I'd managed to fake it quite well, but then they hit me with the news that there were only two places left on the trial, as opposed to the ten that Ed had mentioned the last time I'd seen him; suddenly my fakery vanished into thin air.

I was still crying on the way home. My carer was surprisingly unsympathetic: 'It's like the lottery. You have to be in it to win it, and someone always does. If they'd said you weren't in it – *then* you'd have something to cry about.' I said, 'But nobody wins the lottery.' It seemed like an appropriate metaphor. I had already lost out in the genetic lottery and now, with hopes fading of being one of the few, I wanted someone to empathise with me and accept that this was basically just so much shit. I wish she could simply have said, 'I'm sorry this has happened to you' instead of trying to banish my negative thoughts. The hope of getting on the trial had sustained me through some difficult times and now I had to accept that it was vanishingly unlikely. I felt purposeless, drifting aimlessly from one boring appointment to the next. After a while they all merged into one.

Ed's colleague at the HD clinic saw me when Ed was away. I hadn't realised Ed wasn't going to be there and my disappointment must have been obvious: I was irritable and disinclined to engage with someone I didn't know and might never see again. She had Ed's manner but felt like a poorly executed replica to me. I realised that I'd bonded with him in the years of adversity and we were now friends.

How had that happened? I respected him as a man of science and as a human being, because he never judged. I could tell him everything and he could be trusted with my secrets. Unlike my husband or friends, he knew me inside out (quite literally, on the day we marvelled at an MRI scan of my brain). He said nice things about how my efforts to keep on thinking and writing may have been more neuroprotective than taking fish oil or other supplements every day, as my stepmother had made my father do. No one else in my life was as generous with compliments and he even trusted me with his story, which I was touched by. There were strange parallels where our narratives intersected; he'd even been splitting up with his own partner when Tom left me.

Before I had HD, I used to get melodramatic about scratches and upset stomachs. I had a split nail for years that no medical professional could explain. It hurt quite a bit and I kept catching it on things (I got Murph to pay for an MRI at a private hospital but the results were inconclusive). I was terrified of bugs and made everyone who crossed our threshold sanitise, which was hard to enforce without being rude to guests. I hid from my vomiting children when I should have been helping them.

In my defence, psychosomatic illnesses are no less real if you are suffering inauthentically. I was always misdiagnosing myself and trying to get doctors to agree. I remember feeling outraged when a GP I'd never seen before refused to accept that I had necrotising fasciitis (the flesh-eating virus), and once spent a whole night on the bathroom floor because I was convinced I had food poisoning, even though no one else who'd eaten the same meal had been similarly afflicted. Everyone used to get dragged into these dramas. Now that I've really got something to moan about, no one wants to listen, as their reserves of goodwill were all exhausted by my complaints about the nail.

I printed out my medical records to corroborate my Universal Credit claim but could not physically attach all 370 pages. The notes were hard to read or make sense of. Every interaction was elaborated; a catalogue of woes. It was also a record of my relationships with my doctors, which have been dysfunctional at times and mutually rewarding at others. I have certainly put them through it. I wouldn't have wanted to be in the consulting room with me, always thinking I knew better than they did and then bolting from the room in a huff.

I was surprised to find that I had received my initial HD diagnosis as early as 7 July 2010. I'm writing this in 2019 so it has been nearly ten years, which is quite the marathon. I first attended the HD clinic in Queen's Square in 2014. I was seen by Ed's predecessor, Dr Haider, and Tom came along too, as he always used to (I can picture us arguing on the way there and being stared at by passers-by). Dr Haider's notes say he was pleased to find that the cocktail of drugs prescribed me by an NHS psychologist seemed to be working for my longstanding depression, but 'the issues that brought Charlotte to us at this difficult period in her life were compounded by the fact that Tom was away for work, a driving accident that she suffered while dealing with the children in the car and difficulties relating to her ability to function as well as she wants to at work' (this was the *Feminist Times* era, when I was still pretending I could do as much as my colleagues).

He goes on to explain that HD affects patients' ability to plan and carry out tasks as well as motivation, and suggests reducing my workload, limiting distractions and trying to focus on one task at a time. He emphasises how sustaining a marriage and one's own career while looking after children can be difficult for anyone. Dr Haider notes that I had been verbally aggressive to Anna on more than one occasion, but that we attributed this to stress from the situation I was in (eventually, work gave me up when *Feminist Times* ran out of money).

A little later, he says that he has been contacted by Tom about my sleep problems and restlessness: 'Charlotte wonders whether this might be a form of restless leg syndrome and has suggested benzodiazepine treatment and withdrawal of mirtazapine'. I was diagnosing my own symptoms from a Google search as a transparent ploy to get them to prescribe Valium and, as usual, I wanted immediate action. My GP had refused to give me Valium because she didn't want me to add benzo addiction to my other problems, which seems reasonable now but didn't then. I was a difficult customer and would certainly have complained to the manager if there'd been one.

*

My first encounter with Ed at the HD clinic was fractious because I was annoyed that Dr Haider had left (I really do hate seeing new people!). I may not have been nice to him but at least I didn't think I could do his job better than he could; having finally stopped diagnosing my own symptoms, I left them for him to interpret. I've enjoyed reading the letters he wrote to my GP about me, which chart both the development of the illness and his medical and human responses to my symptoms.

Apart from empathising, Ed had a suggestion to combat apathy that might have worked but would have been hard to enact: like Dan, he thought I should get a dog. Many of his patients had had their quality of life improved by getting a low-maintenance mutt for companionship, and to motivate them to leave the house. This sounded like a great idea, but I knew I'd find it hard to trust the judgement of anything that loved me unconditionally.

As well as prescribing lifestyle shifts and giving me good advice, Ed kept adjusting my medication as the illness progressed. The psychiatrist I'd seen for my depression a few years earlier had prescribed five different pills for my mood and a couple of mood stabilisers for good measure. Ed suggested melatonin for the insomnia; it wasn't licensed by the NHS but they agreed to let me have it in the end, after my GP fought my corner. This came as a nice surprise, as there have been times when Ed has suggested a drug but a GP I don't know has refused to follow his advice. It's more than upsetting when this happens, as GPs aren't HD experts and I inevitably get shirty with them.

When the melatonin didn't work (even at the highest dose), Ed prescribed zopiclone, starting with a low dose and working up to 6.5 over time. I couldn't get an appointment with my usual GP so risked seeing someone else, and instantly regretted it when they said I could only have zopiclone for a week because I would get addicted and it would stop working. As with the melatonin, they said it was out of their hands – they just weren't allowed to prescribe zopiclone long term. Ed intervened and called them to explain his thinking, which I was immensely grateful for. Soon after, my usual GP called me, apologised on behalf of her colleague and said the prescription was waiting to be picked up at the practice. It was a result, but the whole process had felt like a battle, which could only be bad for my health – and even with the zopiclone on board, I still couldn't sleep.

Then, in 2015, Ed introduced olanzapine into the now-quite-crowded cocktail of drugs I was taking. He said it would help with the involuntary movements, as well as the irritability and aggression ... and it did! It also helped me sleep, so things were soon much easier for everyone at home.

We also talked about my reading problems. I'd found it difficult to concentrate on books even before I had HD, but part of me had always suspected that that was probably the books' fault. We'd grown apart, and I hadn't paid much attention – but now that I was on my own all day with nothing to do but drift towards the TV, I wanted them back. Novels could have offered companionship, diversion and, more importantly, an escape route to another world, but they'd shut me out just when I needed them most.

Ed thought this worthy of further investigation, so I had a meeting with a speech and language therapist at the National Hospital to talk it over. I believed I had aphasia, which is common in stroke victims, but Ed hadn't seen that in any of his HD patients. The speech and language therapist ran some tests and said he thought my problem was with semantic skills (or, to make those words easier to understand, understanding what words mean). When Ed saw this report, he said it was probably caused by HD but was certainly 'somewhat unusual'. Then he added, 'It may be of some comfort to know that you're a special case.'

It *was* of some comfort. I had always taken a small measure of satisfaction from the fact that my disease was one that no one had heard of, and now it seemed I was a special case within this already special category! I was amused to find this letter, as it shows how well Ed knows me; it never led to a solution, though. I still can't read but I'm surrounded by books, and keep on buying more. There is no more shelf space for the new ones so they pile up on every available surface, but I refuse to admit defeat and let them go.

If only *specialness* were a criterion for getting on the trial (at least it isn't contraindicated ... ?). Being friends with Ed won't make me any more likely to get on it either. I know it would be unethical, but I wish he could have a word with his manager and plead my case: I have a young family and am not too thin or fat.

I'm ill but not too ill. I'm even sleeping a bit better these days.

For a long time I had regular appointments at the sleep clinic of the Royal National Throat, Nose and Ear Hospital, to try to get to the bottom of my insomnia. In the end they proposed a mandibular splint for my snoring; I no longer shared a bed with Tom so didn't need to stress about keeping him awake, but Ed said the snoring might actually be what was keeping *me* awake. I agreed initially but the splint turned out to be this sort of medieval torture instrument that locked my jaw forward, making me look like Jaws from the James Bond films. It amused the children no end but I couldn't bear the thought of wearing it to bed. It's still on my bedside table now, gathering dust. I could open a museum of medical curiosities with all the unused bits of kit I have lying around.

I wrote a gloomy email to Ed about the fact that there was nothing left to look forward to; the only certainty was future degeneration and ending up like Murph. At his suggestion, and without expecting it to make any difference, I made contact with what I suppose I'm going to have to call 'the HD community'. My local support group only meets a short bus ride away but I'd got out of the habit of going, largely out of apathy. It's run by volunteers, and the coordinator is benign and well informed about the illness. His wife died in 2001 but he's still committed to being there for us.

The meetings were originally held in a community centre, until that became prohibitively expensive; now they're in a café that never has quite enough seats for all of us. It gets too hot in summer, with leatherette diner-style banquettes that our bare legs stick to, and I'm always worried about knocking over my drink, or someone else's. I'm also over-conscious of being over-heard by other customers – our sad stories are hard enough to relate without an additional audience. To mitigate this, the coordinator always quietly mingles and makes sure he has spoken to us all individually.

It took a few months of attending for me to get to know the regulars and feel like I was connecting with them rather than observing at one remove like a jour-nalist. But when I finally started sharing, it was like the emotional floodgates had opened and I didn't care who was listening. I told them everything about everything without editing any of it. I felt comfortable talking to them and was pleased to discover that we had a lot in common, despite us all being at different points on the long walk in the wrong direction that was HD.

One woman told me about her husband, who'd been sectioned and sent to a psychiatric unit where none of the staff had any experience of working with people with HD. He'd just wanted to come home and couldn't understand what he was doing there. I told her about Murph being sent to a home where most of the inmates had dementia, and how I couldn't get over the feeling that I'd let him down by not doing more to rescue him. Another woman had travelled the world and attended dozens of classical concerts, despite being more disabled than me, all while I'd been sat at home staring at the TV.

She was wobbly on her crutches so I was amazed when she said she went everywhere on public transport.

I was pleased to be going to the group, which the old me would have disdained. I started moaning to them instead of Tom, which improved everything at home. I was proud of the new me and pleased when Tom commended me on it; he said he didn't regret his time with me and was grateful to have been part of the story I have related here. It had certainly been a rollercoaster but he was glad he'd bought a ticket.

I emailed Ed to tell him I was feeling less gloomy and he wrote back saying he'd gone to America to present the results from the latest trial, which was why he hadn't been able to see me at the clinic. It was going very well but they were in a 'recruitment pause' while the protocol was rejigged to make it more tolerable for participants. As always, he asked if I had put on weight (they won't be able to enrol me if I'm under 57kg), but he seemed pleased to hear that I'd taken steps to rejig my life.

I'm still waiting to hear if I'm on the trial, which I should be used to by now. It's a cruel irony that HD is making me more impatient exactly when I need to be more Zen; wants feel more like needs and everything seems urgent. I need to adapt to my illness as it evolves and get used to the idea that there will be more losses on the way. The only thing that's certain is that it will get worse, and I will drift further and further away from the person I used to be.

Is my life worth living? I can never decide. My mind is constantly weighing up the pros and cons of carrying on. In the pros column: my interactions with my children. They need me to balance out Tom – everyone needs someone they can feel comfortable moaning to – and tutor them in the ways of Ravenishness. The cons column: I'm jealous of my friends, people in ads, people with dogs, Tom and, yes, my children, which is understandable but unseemly. I hate hearing them talk about going on holiday or out to dinner.

I also hate hearing about other people's professional or romantic successes. When my housemate got a boyfriend, I couldn't bear to hear about him. When Tom takes John back to his flat each evening, I feel like my heart is breaking. The family dinners that seemed like a good idea for the sake of the children didn't work in the end, as I felt inhibited by Tom's presence.

Another con is having to constantly ask people to help me with something – a great big list of somethings that is certain to get longer. I used to be able to manage to wash my hair and all aspects of 'personal care', including putting on sanitary towels, but now I curse those infernal wings that have made an already difficult job impossible. I used to like going to cafés for lunch but now I don't because I spill food on myself or tip over my coffee. The last time I tried it, I kept having to get John to ask them for cloths and kitchen roll, which didn't seem fair. It's all just so embarrassing.

Our stairs are very steep and slippery, so I suppose it was only a matter of time before I twisted my ankle. It looked like the bone in my foot was fractured, which could have meant a special boot or crutches, but eventually the doctor advised me to just go home and keep the foot raised. He was shocked when I said I was regularly negotiating four flights of stairs, and wondered how I would stay safe in the house in future. That tipped the balance: it felt like the house and me just weren't working well together any more. It was time to say goodbye and move on, no matter how hard that was.

I'm fairly sure Tom hadn't been looking forward to our session with the couples' therapist any more than me. We seemed to be locked into the same old familiar, inescapable dynamic in the car on the way there, even though I'd long since acknowledged that I'd been a bad wife for years before the HD symptoms started. By the time we got to the therapist (in Hampstead again, bingo!), it seemed clear that both of us wanted to get out of this tormenting psychodrama rather than fix our marriage, which was probably beyond repair.

I think Tom believed I was going to try to cajole him into coming back to me, but the idea of divorce turned out to be so liberating that I was the one who ended up suggesting it. It was empowering – what a relief. Of course I was sad, but it felt like a good way to finish. I'd finally resolved to sell the house as soon as possible and avoid slagging Tom off in front of the children, which would have been bad for their mental health (and wasn't something I particularly felt like doing anyway). I texted him the next day and said, 'I hope you will want to be my friend even if you don't feel like you have to be. In the future, that is.' He replied, 'I think I will actually.'

A letter from a colleague of Ed's who's in charge of recruitment on the trial told me how competitive it was, trying to manage expectations – I wished I hadn't opened it – but at least Ed assured me that they will certainly give the drug to all of us if it works. Even if I'm not on the trial, there will still be hope for Anna and John.

On that score, I've noticed that both of my children have suddenly stopped moaning about everything because I have, and everyone is suddenly feeling more positive about life because I am; I also have some new carers who were trained by a specialist in brain injury and neurological illness. One of them has even read Stephen Grosz's book, so I am able to discuss it with her at length. She is as calm and quiet as a millpond and the house has never been cleaner or more organised, which means I hardly ever lose things. I've given up all the things I can't afford: drugs, coffee, cigarettes, haircuts, exercise classes. This hasn't affected my quality of life as much as I'd thought it would, and is certainly better than worrying about being in the red. It has taken me more than twenty years to work this out.

As I approach the end of this book, it's striking me that I can't recall anything in it, which is a strange feeling. I'm really proud of it but now I will have nothing to do except watch TV, go to appointments and wait for the children to come home. One of the occupational therapists suggested I should keep a journal but, ultimately, I've never actually found writing that enjoyable. I knew what I was doing when I destroyed the book of doom and didn't blame anyone else for the fact that it was unpublishable.

I wouldn't have been able to do this book if I hadn't collaborated with my brother on it. All my solo projects have been scuppered by perfectionism and hubris. I was so pleased when Dan agreed to help me with this, because it was clearly always going to be a lot more than a simple proofreading job. The process was as important as the end result, and it's made us much closer. As well as being a good editor, he is always able to remember our history and my voice, even when I've struggled to hear it myself. I have been amplified but I haven't drowned him out, which feels miraculous; I'm proud of us both for surviving long enough to complete this impossible task together.

9

The Trial

'Are you sure about this? It's the one thing you didn't want to happen.'

I was standing with my lawyer in the corridor outside a room where Tom and I were still in the middle of a mediation session; she'd asked if she could have a quick word with me alone because I'd just agreed to his plan to sell our house.

Was I sure? I was not. But Tom had already made it clear that he wasn't going to move back in, even though he was now paying through the nose for the two-bedroom flat he was renting up the road as well as the mortgage and bills for the house I was still living in. My proposal had been for us to have our own lives while living under the same roof, which would have solved a lot of problems, but he'd been adamant: if he'd moved back in he would have had to look after both the children and me, and the persistent demands of HD would inevitably have drowned out their needs. I could see what he meant, and it made me feel like a bad mother, but it was HD that had made me unmotherly – I couldn't help not being able to re-member their PE kits or manage the logistics of their lives.

The plan we eventually agreed on was to buy two three-bedroom flats with the money we raised from selling the house. My paid housemate would move in with me and Anna while John went backwards and forwards like *Millie Inbetween*, a CBBC drama about a divorced couple who got on better after they'd split up and their new partners had been seamlessly integrated into newly defined family units. Would this be the case for me and Tom? It was easy enough to imagine him with someone else but I couldn't see that happening for me.

In some ways, a fresh start sounded like a good idea. If I stayed in our old home I would be constantly surrounded by reminders of the arguments we'd had about my extravagant tastes. However much Tom had earned, we'd always been in the red; as long as I was in it, the house would feel like a crime scene where I was perpetrator, victim and witness. Why would I want to stay there?

I also had to admit that the house had become hard for me to manage. There were so many stairs – I'd fallen down them more than once and ended up in A&E. I kept losing things, everything I touched broke, and I could never remember how the Vola taps worked. I felt precarious there and out of sync with the space I used to identify with.

My attachment was not so much to the house as to the life I'd led in it. I missed our all-night parties and the lively kitchen-table debates of the *Feminist Times* era. I wanted to talk to grown-ups but all my new carers seemed to be the same age as Anna, with branded tops and Air Force trainers.

My new twenty-year-old housemate came from a village in East Anglia and was an Ed Sheeran fan. She'd never been to London before so I felt responsible for making sure it worked out for her. She'd arrived with her parents the morning after a party, when the house was still trashed. As the parents were leaving, her mother had said, 'Please look after my baby', which seemed like a lot of responsibility for an ill person to take on – wasn't it supposed to be the other way around? She was really kind, and I was grateful to her for doing carers' tasks when that wasn't what she'd signed up for, but we didn't have much in common.

Tom thought he was being responsible by making sure I had people around but it wasn't the same as having him. I tried to be nice to my new housemate, though, as none of it was her fault and I knew I couldn't expect her to stand in for Tom.

He was going to be in Bristol with his family for Christmas, and he'd made it clear that I wouldn't be welcome. The idea of being anywhere with him and knowing that I wasn't wanted was worse than the prospect of being on my own, but I still felt ambivalent about him. During the mediation session, I'd even started to feel like I didn't want him to come back after all – he was too strict and always made me eat my greens, and I couldn't be myself in front of him.

*

The HD drug trial had receded from view. After years of holding my breath and hoping that I'd make it on to the distant and ever-diminishing longlist for the trial, it only seemed to be getting further away. Every time I went to the hospital I could sense them managing my expectations. And then that Enroll-HD doctor explained to me there were only two places on the trial and thousands of people competing for them, so I told myself I should be realistic about my chances and assume I wouldn't get one.

To protect myself from this crushing disappointment, I imposed an information blackout and stopped googling 'HD drug trial'. I didn't read any updates on the HDBuzz website, which I used to check regularly, or go to my support group in case they discussed it. I felt left out and resentful of the four fortunates whom fate had selected to be part of this era-defining journey. I was sure that they were all highly deserving, but at the same time equally sure that I was rather more so.

The destination may have been uncertain but I wanted to be on the bus, with Ed and his colleagues sitting alongside me. Annoyingly, people kept telling me that I had to be a shoo-in for the trial because I was a friend of Ed's; I'd have to explain that medical trials were not like nightclubs, with a VIP area for people with connections. I was sending weekly prompts to Ed for updates about when and how they would start recruiting for the trial, but worried that this chivvying might prove counterproductive: being irritating might well be one of the many contraindications for getting on the longlist.

By this time I'd worked out how to live with my limitations and see HD as a learning tool for life, but it was still difficult, with as many bleak days as good ones. Thinking about the future was dangerous as I kept picturing myself being carted off to a local authority home with no specialist HD staff because there was no money to pay for anything nicer. The trial would have given me a sense of purpose; without it I felt directionless. The dull days all merged into one another. When my carers left I'd just lie in bed for hours, exhausted but unable to sleep – wired by caffeine, nicotine and anxiety. I forgave myself for taking up everything bad for me again, as there was nothing else to do – I still struggled with boredom and could not read. I hope the reader will forgive me too. My mind is always stuck on the same subject, which is what HD doctors call perseverative thinking. Although I was never addicted, even small units seemed to make this facet of my mental landscape worse.

I'd wait for the children to come home, looking forward to seeing them, but unlike me they had social lives so they'd usually just go straight out again. John said, 'You need a hobby, Mum', and he may have been right, but what could I do? Everyone seemed to think that gardening would have been good for my mental health, but to me it looked too much like hard work (a friend of mine once said that it was 'like doing housework outdoors', which John thought was hilarious). There was nothing to do and nothing to look forward to, and the only certainty was that I would decline and fall like

Murph and my grandmother. Every tomorrow would be worse than every today.

I was so used to getting bad news that my first reaction to the email from Ed inviting me to be screened for the 'Gen-PEAK' trial was disbelief. I'd never heard of it, for one thing – the wonder drug trial I'd been trying to get on to was called 'Gen Extend'. The last time I'd seen Ed he'd said that there were trials within trials that I might be eligible for, but of course I'd forgotten about that. I read the email over and over again, and sent it to everyone in case I was misinterpreting it.

When I emailed Ed to ask if he meant what I thought he meant, his reply was an unambiguous yes. That's when I started getting excited. He was a responsible doctor and wouldn't have given me hope unless it was likely, if not certain, that I'd meet the inclusion criteria for the trial. I was delighted to learn that I could end up being 'Patient 1' on this investigational branch of the main trial, where the effects of the new huntingtin-protein-lowering drug on blood, spinal fluid and urine before and after dosing would help them determine how, when and in what dose to administer it in the future. The invitation made me feel very important, a genetic pioneer.

The drug had apparently surpassed the doctors' expectations when they'd tested it on mice with HD. Some of the mice had even got slightly better, which seemed miraculous, and they knew it was safe to use on humans because they'd already tried it on a brave cohort upon whom it had had no significant side effects. The second phase of the trial was about efficacy but they knew they were in the right ballpark with the right drug.

They sent me information sheets explaining what would happen and when. The first step would be a screening day where they'd check that I was a good fit for the trial. I asked Ed if it would be sensible to go to a festival the weekend before this screening but he said no – I'd need to be 'match fit', with no illegal drugs in my system. I'd also need to be fatter than I'd ever been to reach the target weight of 57kg. I had always been thin but was, by this time, even more so than usual as HD tends to make people lose weight.

This was the first challenge and I took it very seriously, buying a set of scales for the first time ever and weighing myself every couple of days. I find eating really boring so it was a chore, but I got there in the end with a couple of days to spare. Anna and my housemate were dismayed to find that they too had put on weight following the regimen of junk food, milkshakes and cakes that I'd subjected them to.

I was told to expect blood tests to measure my general health, check the status of the illness and monitor how the medication was working in my body. There would be neurological exams and scrutiny of my medical history and existing conditions, including hospitalisations. The history of my HD over the past two years would be explored, as well as my past and current use of illegal drugs.

I wondered if cannabis oil counted; I'd been taking it for my insomnia every night for a year and it had been transformative. A friend had smuggled some in from

Jamaica for me. When I first took it I felt wired rather than relaxed, but then I adjusted the dose and took it only in the evenings instead of three times a day. I was amazed and delighted to find myself falling asleep on the sofa every night and having to haul myself up to bed. CBD oil was the legal version but I'd already tried it without success.

I couldn't decide if I should tell Ed about the cannabis oil and possibly rule myself out of the trial, but I assumed CBD oil would be okay so I told him I was taking that instead. He replied quickly and said CBD oil was fine, then emailed again a few days later with an urgent update from the drug company, who'd said that taking CBD oil would disqualify me from the trial. I was disappointed and couldn't think what else I could use that would work as well. My carer suggested camomile tea, which really annoyed me – I'd already tried herbal tea and 'sleep hygiene' but no strategy was a match for the endless HD dance that convulsed my body every night.

The screening day was intense and exhausting. Tom was there as he had eventually agreed to be my trial companion (let's steer clear of 'buddy' for now), supporting me and also helping them by monitoring how the drug affected me if we made it through screening to dosing. I was nervous – the prospect of being a lab rat was daunting, however grateful I was for the opportunity.

The minute we arrived at the Leonard Wolfson Experimental Neurology Centre on the ground floor of the UCL Queen Square Institute of Neurology, they asked if

I could be pregnant. I told them I hadn't had sex for six years but they still insisted on doing a pregnancy test. There were blood and heart rate tests and my BMI was calculated; Ed high-fived me when we found that I had hit my target weight (just).

Then there were neurological and cognitive assessments, as well as some more personal questions. When they asked if I'd ever taken illegal drugs I assured them I hadn't. I was worried that the cocaine I'd taken two weeks earlier would still be detectable in my blood, although Decca had assured me that it only stayed in your system for three days.

There was a good vibe at the centre – I think they were just happy to finally be testing something they thought might work as opposed to something they knew wouldn't (Ed once told me that they'd even tested fish oil to see if it was neuroprotective, as people were claiming on the internet; it wasn't). They asked me if I'd had any suicidal thoughts, and I was pleased to answer truthfully that I hadn't for ages. I wasn't a glass-half-full person yet but felt myself edging towards that. My life was suddenly laced with hope.

After the screening day I waited anxiously to hear from Ed about whether I'd made it through the *X-Factor*-style auditions and secured my place in the live final, when the world would be watching. He kept saying that the nurses would tell me if I'd made it but I badgered him anyway, texting him compulsively.

It took three weeks for the results of the blood tests to come through. They confirmed that I didn't have cancer,

AIDS or diabetes but I did have deformed HD DNA. Ed emailed to say, 'It is overwhelmingly likely that you will get on this trial.' And I did!

Then something strange happened. All my friends thought I should be happy now that I finally had what I wanted – what everyone with HD wanted. They stopped visiting so my therapist was the only person I could talk to, and I couldn't afford to pay him. Even Dan was unsympathetic and thought I should just be grateful to be on the trial. No one seemed to be considering the fact that the drug wasn't actually a cure and I still had a horrible illness. And Gen-PEAK was clearly not going to be a walk in the park.

The plan for the next few months looked daunting and scary. I hate injections and blood tests. They were planning to admit me for a 'treatment period' of a week. I would receive two doses of the protein-lowering drug and this would be administered by a catheter rather than a lumbar puncture. On day one of the treatment period they were going to speed through a whole range of procedures: urine collection, neurological examination, ECG, halter ECG, cerebral spinal fluid collection, blood tests, investigational therapy. Dosing would be on day two.

On the screening day, the nurse had said they wouldn't let me embark on this process unless I had someone to take me to my appointments and pick me up. Tom was falling out of view, as I'd feared he might, but now Anna said she would come and get me when she could, if it was after school. She found it all very interesting so I didn't feel like I was imposing on her, and she was happy to commit to visiting me when I became an in-patient as well. Anna was empathic and reliable, a perfect trial companion; I knew she would answer any SOS texts speedily and check in regularly. And I wouldn't have to worry about looking after her – some of the other candidates for the role were phobic about hospitals, and Tom fainted at the sight of blood.

But I was still lonely and increasingly isolated. I tried to talk to my carers and housemate about my predicament but they were too young to impart any wisdom, apart from urging me to stop worrying about everything. They were always laughing at YouTube videos of animals and showing them to me, which was torture – didn't they realise I couldn't even smile?

One of my best friends asked if she could read this book, but as we were on holiday at the time I couldn't show it to her myself. When I asked Dan to email it to me, he did so with the prescient footnote, 'Hope she likes it, but don't take any notice if she doesn't!' She ended up declaring it unpublishable, and I was devastated. Writing the book and trying to get it published had been the driving force of my life for nearly a year, so it felt horribly wrenching to be suddenly convinced that the whole thing was pointless.

Once again I found myself thinking about suicide – drawing up a pros and cons list for life. Should I keep on keeping on, knowing that I would never get better, or end it while I still could? Without sex or ideas (or hobbies), the future looked bleak. Anna and John were in the pros list but I had to balance how terrible it would be for them if I took the Dignitas route against how terrible it would be if I didn't.

This was the biggest decision of my life but I was ill equipped to make it, and time was running out: I couldn't put it off, kick the can down the road and reassess in a couple of years, because that might be too late. I wasn't sure how much my mind would have deteriorated by then but I knew the rules. Even the Swiss would baulk at putting me to sleep if I didn't have the capacity to consent, which I had then but wouldn't for long.

I'd got as far as joining Dignitas and starting to assemble the comprehensive medical records they'd need to support my application when two important things changed. First, the book that I had thought unpublishable turned out not to be – we found a proper publisher with an editor who loved what I'd written so far. And then I got an email from Ed that included the words, 'If you make it through Gen-PEAK, Gen Extend awaits.' The open-label drug trial that had been on the news was at last in sight. Why was I in this privileged position? I didn't want to ask in case they changed their minds.

I wasn't looking forward to being in hospital for a week for the first phase of the Gen-PEAK trial, though. I was going to be there for my fiftieth birthday, being prodded and dosed and having bits of myself drained away. It was certainly going to be a lot more memorable than the party I'd have thrown otherwise.

*

The trial protocol meant that everything had to run on time, but the doctors and nurses at the Leonard Wolfson Centre were careful not to stress me out. I arrived at 8 a.m. on the Monday and was whisked away to Room 2 for the first of a hundred assessments that I would soon get bored with but seemed novel on the first day. They put the ECG halter on and said I'd need to wear it at all times, all week.

There was a TV in Room 2 but it wasn't working. I panicked as this felt like a necessity, not a luxury (I was always glued to the news channel at home, but often wondered whether the content was making this an anxiety-inducing activity rather than a soothing one). I didn't have an iPad and the screen on my phone was too small to see. What could I do to distract myself from what was going on?

Ed's colleague, a softly spoken Portuguese man, appeared occasionally to perform neurological tests on me. He made me walk up and down the corridor heel-to-toe, tested my reflexes with a hammer and pricked me with a needle to see if I could feel the difference between blunt and sharp. These tests were more annoying than invasive but I never got used to the blood tests, which seemed to happen every five minutes.

A nervous nurse repeatedly failed to insert a cannula into my left arm so they could take blood every two hours, and tried to distract me from the pain she was inflicting by talking about mindfulness. I felt sorry for her and bad about asking her more competent colleague, a former cancer nurse who'd boasted that she could 'put cannulas in in my sleep', to take over. She was garrulous and gave a running commentary on what she was doing, as well as telling me what to expect from the trial and urging me to drink lots of water, as they were intending to test my pee every few hours.

When I did go to the toilet, it was difficult not to get tangled up in the strings of the ECG monitor – the more things they attached to me, the harder it was to man-oeuvre. In preparation for dosing, a neurological surgeon I hadn't met before put a catheter in that snaked up my back like a goth tattoo. There was a tap at the top, on my shoulder, through which they going to 'milk' me for cerebral spinal fluid every few hours. Ed told me he was going to stay for two nights in a room down the cor-ridor and do the CSF collection himself, which made me feel honoured. The nurses seemed surprised that a con-sultant would commit to a sleepover.

Our relationship was hard to define: we were friends and collaborators heading off on an adventure together but neither of us knew the way. I genuinely loved him! Unlike other consultants I'd met, he never patronised me or made me feel like he knew more about my illness than I did. I felt like I could tell him anything and he'd listen without judging me. He'd witnessed my HD story as it had unfolded over the years and been a consistent presence in my life who'd always had my back when other people let me down. I felt as close to him as I did to my children.

On dosing day, I was exhausted because of the night before – they'd woken me up every two hours to take blood and CSF. At 11.43 they gave me the first dose through the catheter. They told me to get out of bed and walk up and down the corridor, which made me feel sick but was necessary to make sure the drug got to my brain instead of hanging around my spine. We discussed my expectations in case they were unrealistic, but they weren't. I knew it wasn't going to be a quick fix but I was playing a long game by then. I had finally learned to be patient.

At some point a woman from the drug company appeared with a gift for me in a cool box labelled with my name and trial number: it was official! Then, as an early birthday present, Ed brought in the contract for the book that we were collaborating on to sign. I couldn't have been prouder.

The night I turned fifty felt momentous. Even as it was happening I was aware that it would make a great ending for this book and worried about not being able to remember it (Ed has suggested voice memos but I can't stand the sound of my own voice). The TV still didn't work but they'd managed to get Radio 4 on my laptop, so I was plugged into the news. I felt shit, but in a way that was oddly familiar: it was another drug hangover, but this time from something that was meant to be in me. Ed was my dealer! The drug he'd given me was no less of a gamble than an illegal one as they didn't know what it was going to do.

At 5 a.m. he came into my room with a Waitrose cheesecake that had candles on it and another present: the packet that the drug they'd given me had come in, which proved I was Patient 001.

They moved me into a room in the private wing of the hospital. There was a working TV and the food was better, but it felt a bit impersonal after all the noise and bustle of Room 2. I had lots of visitors and they all brought food – I'd said the food was rubbish when I was in Room 2 but now it was all fine dining in the private ward and the message hadn't got through. Murph's friend Julian brought a shopping bag full of snacks and ready meals.

After a while every surface was covered in food, and I was starting to feel hemmed in by it. I felt duty-bound to try to work my way through it, though – Tom would have told me off if I'd asked them to remove or bin it. I was missing cigarettes so I snacked instead of smoking, which was difficult to accomplish from my position propped up on the bed, not quite high enough to reach the tray table. My room felt cluttered and messy with clothes all over the floor, just like it always did at home. I'd only been there for a couple of hours.

Tom's sister Frances arrived with sunflowers, which I was pleased about as I wasn't expected to eat them. Her presence was soothing but I didn't feel much like talking – I had a terrible headache, which Ed had told me to expect, but it was more than disagreeable even when I was prepared for it. It only went away when I lay down flat, and then not for very long.

But still I kept on eating. There was sea bass for dinner and I had truffles with Ed's cake for dessert. I tried to go to sleep but it just wouldn't happen; I kept summoning the night nurse to change the bed position but, really, I just wanted someone to talk to. At about 2 a.m. I threw up, which gave me a fright. Ed hadn't mentioned vomiting as a side effect and I wasn't sure what to attribute it to. They paged his colleague for advice but he'd turned his phone off, so I continued to panic until I'd done an audit of everything that had passed my lips that day – at which point the whole thing seemed suddenly explicable.

The rest of the week passed without incident. I didn't feel very well but that was only to be expected. They were still taking CSF and blood but the intervals were getting longer, with more time to rest and watch the news. The headaches came and went.

Every day they took something off: the ECG halter went first, then the cannula. The day before I was due to be discharged, they took off the catheter, and suddenly I didn't feel like a lab rat any more. Ed asked me to describe my experience of Gen-PEAK, as they were intending to screen a few more people; I summed it up as 'intense and exhausting but worth it'.

On the last day I was delighted to be free, and proud of myself for making it to the end of the most difficult phase of Gen-PEAK (there would be more appointments but I wouldn't have to stay in hospital for them). Ed said the sponsor was pleased with how it had gone and wanted to take a picture of us both that we could use in this book, but I wouldn't let him as I wasn't looking my best.

The hospital bedding had been sweaty so I was really looking forward to getting back to my high-thread-count Egyptian cotton linen. Tom came to get me and, just as I'd expected, he put all the uneaten snacks and ready meals from the fridge into a plastic bag and took them home with him. I was pleased to be going but felt I was going to miss everyone, and a thank-you seemed inadequate. They'd treated me like a princess.

Ed had predicted that I'd sleep for two days as soon as I got home, and that's pretty much what happened. As I got ready to go to bed that night I was on my own again, feeling drained and sad. But then Anna came back and we went through our 'best bits' from my time on the trial, like they do on reality shows. We had some funny stories to relate, and she was as pleased as me that I'd made it through the first part of Gen-PEAK intact.

After taking a few days to regenerate, I thought it would be nice to have a birthday party after all. The guests of honour would be Ed and his fiancé, who I'd heard a lot about, and although they both quickly accepted the invitation I was almost hoping they wouldn't come – I couldn't stand the thought of letting myself down in front of such high-calibre guests.

There was also confusion about the party concept I was going for, so people kept texting for clarification. My previous housemate Lucy had sourced a great image from the internet of a raven wearing Day-Glo headphones under the slogan, 'KEEP ON RAVEN', and I'd used this for the invitations. Everyone I'd sent one to thought I was planning an all-night party with no kids or nibbles, which is what I'd have liked it to be. But I couldn't take drugs because of the trial, so there was no reason not to have children there – nothing was going to happen that I wouldn't have wanted them to see, sadly.

As there would be no drugs, there was no reason not to have food. I delegated this task to Tom and was grateful that he made light work of it. The turnout was better than I'd expected and, as the conversation flowed, I felt like I was starting to remember who I was – I'd missed this.

Everyone seemed to be having a nice time. It was shaping up very well and I wasn't even missing the drugs. Ed and his partner arrived at this optimal point, and the first thing he said to me was, 'How *are* you?' in his HD clinic voice. We talked about the headaches. I was surprised to hear that the HD drug was still in my system and would be for six weeks. Ed told me how pleased he was with what he'd read of my chapters and said he was looking forward to seeing how this last one turned out.

When he was sitting down with a low-alcohol beer, I asked him to explain why he'd decided to become an HD specialist and tell me some of the backstory, clinical and personal, that had set the scene for the trial. He also talked about the Gen-PEAK trial and, prompted by me, related some funny stories from my time as a lab rat in his charge. His fiancé was charming and younger than we'd expected. They left before the party degenerated in the way I'd hoped it might but feared it wouldn't without coke.

The next big thing on the Gen-PEAK schedule was the second dose of the protein-lowering drug – this would be administered through a lumbar puncture, which was going to hurt more than the catheter. My carer took me to the hospital in an Uber, as I had to be

there at 8 a.m. and have the dreaded cannula put in
again so they could take blood four times during the
day. I was used to the neurological exams, which they
always did in the same order. Nothing had changed
since the last time they'd done them.

Disappointingly, the first blood test results were
delayed, throwing their schedule off and propelling me
into an anxious state where I thought that the dosing
might not happen at all. I was back in Room 2 with a
new Spanish doctor who told me Ed had sent a hug,
which I was pleased to receive. The blood results finally
arrived in the nick of time and I was cleared for dosing.
The nurses tried to put me in the right position – lying
on my side with a pillow between my legs – but the cannula kept getting in the way. We got there in the end,
though, and I was presented correctly so that they could
see what they were doing. I just needed to keep still, although this was easier said than done.

They always apologised for hurting me before they
did it and explained exactly what was going to happen.
The nurses would say, 'Sharp scratch' when they were
taking blood (which was more or less true depending on
who was doing it), and I trusted the doctor to be straight
with me. He cleaned my back and injected an anaes-
thetic into the base of my spine before administering the
drug. It was all over in the blink of an eye, and then they
were urging me to get out of bed.

They made me walk up and down the corridor in
my hospital gown as they had before. There weren't
many people there, fortunately, but those twenty

minutes felt like a long time. I started feeling dizzy and sick so I had to lie down again.

At the end of the day, my housemate came to get me. I was pleased to be going home but, instead of going straight back, I thought it would be a good idea to get the Tube from Russell Square to Oxford Circus and go to the shops. I'd just received £900 for taking part in the trial and wanted to blow it irresponsibly, all at once and as soon as possible. And I knew just where I should go to do this: I'd had my eye on a few things that weren't in the sale on the All Saints website, but Anna had discouraged me because she thought I was too old to carry them off. No one could tell me off for spending my money *now* ...

As we got off the Tube and started walking down Regent Street, it struck me that I may have been making a huge mistake. Arm-in-arm with my housemate, I walked as slowly as I could while people crashed into me. Everything hurt but I persevered. We made it to All Saints and I spotted the top I'd seen on their website – it was slightly cropped but I thought it would be okay with high-waisted jeans. My housemate said she thought it would suit me, which I took as a sign even though she was always nice about everything. No sooner had it gone in the basket than I saw a winter coat that would have gone with pretty much anything.

Ten minutes later we were heading to the till with five items, and I'd be embarrassed to say how much it all came to. The bus stop was miles away so we hailed a taxi; I couldn't remember my address but my housemate could. We were stuck in traffic for hours while my discomfort morphed into a subtle but persistent and generalised pain.

When we got back I realised I'd left the receipt in the cab, and felt like crying as I was going to be stuck with these ill-advised purchases. I took them all up to my bedroom and tried them on with my housemate, who assured me that I didn't look like mutton dressed as lamb in the crop top, but I did – it was shorter than I'd expected and left a couple of inches of midriff exposed. The skinny jeans I'd bought didn't fit – the first time I pulled them up, the denim ripped. The hard-to-care-for jumper looked nice enough but I was immediately worried that I'd shrink it even if I followed the washing instructions (this has happened before). I was cross with myself for wasting all that money – it was as if everything I'd learned about budgeting and careful husbandry of my finances over the years had been overturned. I felt like I was back to square one.

For the next few days my legs hurt, and I didn't know whether this was down to the shopping trip or a side effect they hadn't warned me about. I called the trial nurse, who said it was unusual and asked me to come in for an assessment that afternoon. After examining me, the doctor said that headaches were common but my other symptoms were unusual and unaccountable. I confessed to the shopping trip and he was amused rather than disapproving, which I was relieved about.

He thought it would be sensible to do an MRI scan on my spine, even though he didn't think it would show anything. It didn't, but they gave me a CD with the image on it to take away as a souvenir. Anna downloaded it, then set it as the screensaver on my phone; the curved stack of bones looks really beautiful, like a Jenga tower designed by Gaudi. The leg pain went away in a day or so.

At the time of writing I have four trial appointments left to go in my conquest of Gen-PEAK. There is to be no more dosing, just surveillance of blood and CSF for a few months until I'm signed off. Dan came to visit and said I didn't look any worse than the last time he was here, which was encouraging. Everyone wants to know if I'm feeling any better but I can't really tell – I refer them to Ed, who has spoken to me at length about his expectations for the trial. According to him, the best case scenario is that the drug will stop the illness or slow it down; the worst is that it simply won't work.

I want to ask him a question that he probably won't be able to answer. My life is shit – why would I want to prolong it? I've discussed this with Dan, who suggested, controversially, that I could and should learn to be more independent and stop asking people to do things I am perfectly capable of. I used to make him get me things and do my bidding when I was a tyrannical child/teenager – now I make John run up and down two flights of stairs to get me a tissue, and he looks after me rather than the other way around (because he's so young he is malleable, and I'm ashamed to say I take advantage of that). But Anna won't look for my phone even if I offer to pay her, and making Tom do things he didn't want to was, of course, a significant factor in the breakdown of our marriage.

I've never really been independent so I want to give it a go – it would be good for my relationships if I wasn't exploiting anyone but 'working with them', and I wouldn't feel so guilty if I changed my own TV channels and made my own cups of tea. Making a four-course meal may not be a realistic ambition but many small tasks are bound to be achievable. This is all new to me; in the past, my to-do lists invariably referred to things I wanted other people to do while I did something more worthwhile.

I just need to think about things differently. I have become housebound even though I can walk, and stranded on my sofa in front of the TV without knowing why or what to do about it. Selling the house and extensively decluttering will be necessary if I am to have any hope of finding a way of life where my sense of who I am isn't dependent on my Pugin Room wallpaper. Speaking to my lawyer before the second mediation session, I realised that I wanted to sell the house just as much as Tom. The prospect of starting a new chapter is both exciting and scary, but mostly the former.

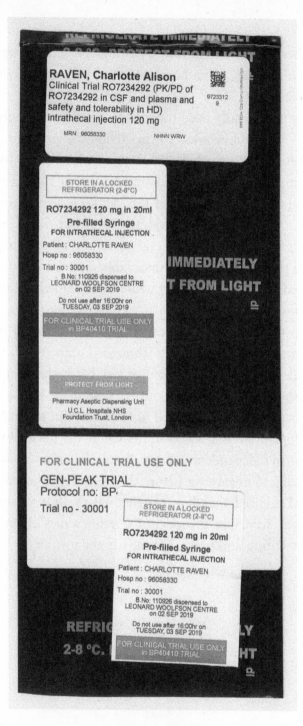

The drug bag

Epilogue
The real ending

On 23 March 2021, Ed Wild rang me. When I asked him how he was, he said, 'Shit – because I've got something terrible to tell you.'

The news was that Roche, the pharmaceutical company conducting the drug trials, had decided to stop treatments. The experimental therapy that was meant to reduce production of the huntingtin protein wasn't working, so there was no point in continuing. The decision was made on the advice of an independent monitoring board so, at the time of writing, we don't know all the details. But the drug definitely hasn't stopped or even slowed the progression of the disease.

The world ended again; it felt exactly the same as the moment of my original diagnosis. Ever since I'd been picked to be on the trial, I'd woken up every morning thinking about the drug. It was like being in love. It was what I needed, wanted, looked forward to. Now that pinprick of light had been blacked out.

I thought of the pain I'd gone through at the hospital in the Gen-PEAK era, when I was an in-patient for a week having CSF taken every hour, the sickness and the headaches. I'd found it all strangely enjoyable because I like to have people constantly focused on me, but it had also given me purpose when little else did.

I've never been afraid to pass on bad news, so I started telling my friends and family. First I explained it to the agency carer, who'd been with me when Ed rang. She suggested I did some breathing exercises, but instead I smoked two cigarettes, one after the other. My carers are competent but not emotionally equipped to deal with a loss like this, and I know I can't expect them to be.

Tom came round after work and made me a big gin and tonic. When John, who has been learning sign language, came back from school, he made the sign for 'I'm sorry'. Then he sat in my lap, and the warmth and weight of him reminded me how much I still need physical human contact. I have always told my children that if they do have HD there will be a treatment by the time they need it. I may need to revise that. All my friends and family empathise when they hear, but they can't be me. I feel lonelier than ever.

After he'd explained to me that the trial was a failure, Ed told me he'd become a star – he's one of the doctors on the public health posters around Camden promoting the Covid-19 vaccination. His life goes on.

Of course, losing my happy ending means that I now also know with absolute certainty what the real ending will be. I will suffer like my father. I will end up in a care home. But what terrifies me most is the thought that no one will want to publish my book now – that somehow the drug trial failure will make my story obsolete. If there's no book, there'll be no true record of who I was. My old ambition persists: I want to be read. I want to be someone, without fucking it up. But it may already be too late.

At least I have one victory. I was determined not to write a misery memoir and, well, I've certainly managed that. No one has triumphed over personal adversity. No one has learned a lesson. No one has learned anything at all.

Friends often used to tell me that even if the new drug therapy didn't work for me, the results from the tests could help future generations of HD sufferers – and now I'm telling myself that too, because it's all I have left. Gen-PEAK may have turned out to be a blind alley but it was still a step on the journey towards a cure, and I still feel proud to have been part of it. I've lived a fairly selfish life in lots of ways, never really wanting to help other people unless there was something in it for me, so it seems oddly fitting that this last thing I did to save myself might end up saving others instead.

Perhaps I do still have some empathy after all.

Afterword
by Professor Ed Wild

As a junior doctor, I had only a general sense I wanted to 'do neurology' because it was clever and had easy night shifts. I'd never met a patient with Huntington's disease, but all doctors have at least heard of it, because it always comes up at medical school, and it tends to stick in the memory. The description of the disease as it currently stood was as not just bad but 'devastating', not just progressive but 'insidious'. Yet the discovery of the gene that causes Huntington's in the 1990s had been heralded as a new era for genetically-powered neuroscience research, and we were assured that it would not be long until this discovery was converted into treatments and cures.

I remember the first time I attended a Huntington's disease multidisciplinary clinic. I met several people considering having the genetic test to determine if they had Huntington's. It was hard to witness: three hours of ruined dreams, of careers abandoned, of daily falls and injuries from dropped irons or frying pans; of husbands and wives who couldn't cope with the daily reality of being shouted at by the person they loved, and eventually left.

It was difficult, but to my amazement it was not depressing. The magic ingredient was research. Interwoven with clinical care was the opportunity for the patients to volunteer to take part in the biggest Huntington's research programme in the UK. Nearly all the patients were keen to do so, from giving blood samples to putting themselves through brain scans, thinking tests and clinical trials of new drugs. In almost every case, they signed up knowing it was unlikely the research would benefit them directly – they wanted to do it so that their kids would grow up in a reality different from their own, or to help their brothers and sisters, nieces or nephews. Many patients had been told before 'there's nothing that can be done' and had resigned themselves to a life being pursued powerlessly by this unassailable foe. But to sign up to take part in the research was to turn round and fight anyway – in the hope of finding a weakness in the armour of Huntington's, in order to save other people from the same fate.

And so I decided I would commit the next three years of my life to researching and treating Huntington's disease. I thought I could probably cope with the messiness and chaos in return for becoming the guy who could walk alongside people in their darkest hour and offer them not only a life raft but also the chance to work together to make a better future. Some seventeen years later, I am a consultant neurologist running a research team at the University College London Huntington's Disease Centre, and have been privileged to be involved in developing and testing some of the most cutting-edge experimental treatments for HD, as well as seeing patients in the National Hospital's HD clinic.

When I saw that she had been allocated to my clinic list for the first time, I already knew *of* Charlotte Raven, from a strange combination of our multidisciplinary team discussions and her public reputation: writer, journalist, thinker. Editor of *Feminist Times*. Early manifest Huntington's disease. Struggling to come to terms with subtle loss of cognitive function. My regular Google News alerts for 'Huntington's disease' had brought her further into my consciousness as the author of such *Guardian* articles as 'Should I take my own life?' and 'I see myself as a recovering narcissist'.

Discovering that this person was now going to be seeing me in the Huntington's clinic was honestly terrifying. As a doctor, it's often strangely aversive to interact with ultra-smart patients. They often want a 'why' far beyond what I can provide, leaving me feeling inadequate. In short, they are harder to impress. A little cognitive decline makes a massive difference to someone whose superior intellect is their life and work; the early Huntington's combination of anxiety, low mood and irritability made me fear an awkward, dispiriting verbal fencing match with a cantankerous intellectual who wouldn't believe a word I told her, and would then write about how crap I was in the *Guardian*.

Despite these misgivings – unimportant in retrospect – being Charlotte's neurologist has always been enjoyable, though I won't say it has ever been easy. In

2016 she told me she was separating from her husband Tom. By coincidence, my seventeen-year relationship had recently ended, in similarly painful but amicable fashion. Neither of us knew what to do next. We talked about the emptiness of it, and the things we'd been doing to distract ourselves. We agreed to let each other know if we found anything that helped. This moment of shared loss and vulnerability stripped away the asymmetry of the circumstances that had brought us together. Nowadays I don't even mind when she teases me – affectionately, I hope – in the national press.

Charlotte's story is a potent reminder of the unpredictability of Huntington's, in spite of its being written in the genes. Even affected siblings can present and progress in wildly different ways. Loss of empathy and self-awareness is a general rule in HD, but Charlotte demonstrates that it need not be inevitable. Huntington's can turn a person into an oil tanker that's lost the ability to steer: its course can be deflected, but it takes the combined force of many small tugboats all pulling in the same direction to make a difference. These can take the form of medications applied judiciously and continuously tweaked as things change, an affable neurologist, a professional carer who shares your taste in music, frank advice from friends, the help of a counsellor, or a sensational Vera Wang dress worn defiantly on your fiftieth birthday. The trick is to assemble a team around you while your brain is in good shape, and then allow them to guide your course once the steering starts to play up. Charlotte judges her pre-HD self harshly, but her later embracing of 'radical empathy' is possible because her earlier self *was* able to assemble a team that, when the time came, was capable of helping her navigate to a tolerable new normal.

Perhaps the most obvious feature of Huntington's disease is the fidgety, dance-like movements known as chorea. The word is Greek – χορεια, a dance – our word 'choreography' is from the same root. Present in most patients with Huntington's, these movements are so distinctive that for most of the time since it was named, the disease was known as Huntington's chorea. This *danse fatale* begins with a very subtle exaggeration of our normal subconscious movements and gestures – a shrug, a flick of the hair, a smile, a crossing of the legs – until these movements get bigger and more frequent, eventually fusing into a continuous flurry of bizarre, twisting, restless writhing and grimacing. Later I coined the Ed Wild 'Tube Test' to help doctors new to Huntington's decide whether someone they saw in clinic has chorea or has just drunk too many coffees: imagine you're sitting opposite the person on the London Underground; if you'd notice their movements and think they had Huntington's in that context, then they probably do.

A curious feature of Huntington's is that a person can have chorea so badly, so obvious that the entire Tube carriage would notice, but they themselves remain blissfully unaware that they are moving abnormally. You can show a Huntington's patient a video of themselves in which they are unidentifiable, and they will say 'that person has HD', but if they recognise themselves in the video they will say 'that's me and the video doesn't show any abnormal movements'. This sounds like denial, but in most cases it's a hardware issue: the connections between the surface of the brain and its deep movement-control structures – the cortex and basal ganglia – gradually disintegrate in Huntington's, producing a curious combination of chorea, and a loss of the ability to sense that one's body is moving uncontrollably. This loss of insight is one of the cruellest features of Huntington's for clinicians and loved ones alike: a person might be entirely helpable, if only they realised how sick they were.

At some point in the 1960s or 70s, it dawned on doctors that this chorea, while obvious, was in fact far from the most disabling feature of Huntington's. Most suffering in Huntington's disease comes from the loss of self: a form of dementia caused by that same accelerated death of neurons. Physicians casually describe this as a combination of cognitive decline, behavioural difficulties and personality change. The reality, as Charlotte has related, is much more messy. This is why we don't call it Huntington's chorea any more. Nowadays it is widely understood that the complex mess that Huntington's creates can only begin to be disentangled by a whole team of neurologists, psychiatrists, specialist nurses and a gaggle of therapists for physical, occupational and speech-and-language needs.

We still get a fair few referral letters from general practitioners mentioning 'Huntington's chorea' or, worse still, 'Huntingdon's chorea'. These are useful pointers that the GP hasn't even googled the disease, often indicating that things for the patient will be particularly grim. Hunting*don* is a town in Cambridgeshire, the constituency of former Prime Minister John Major. Hunting*ton* was the surname of a newly qualified family doctor in New England called George, who was just twenty-two when in 1872 he published his first and only notable paper, 'On Chorea'. In it, he described 'a medical curiosity': a number of cases where a 'dancing propensity' ran in families. 'It is spoken of,' he noted grimly, 'by those in whose veins the seeds of the disease are known to exist, with a kind of horror, and not at all alluded to except through dire necessity, when it is mentioned as "that disorder".'

Huntington's paper was short, but evocative and comprehensive. It gave a pretty good description of how the disease runs in families: 'One or more of the offspring almost invariably suffer from the disease, if they live to adult age. But if by any chance these children go through life without it, the thread is broken and the grandchildren and great-grandchildren of the original shakers may rest assured that they are free from the disease.' We now call this pattern 'autosomal dominant'.

For Huntington's patients, this genetic misfortune has been coupled with centuries of stigma, secrecy, shame, and even persecution. As late as the 1960s, eminent neurologists in the UK were still calling for sterilisation of Huntington's disease patients. It was 121 years after George Huntington's paper that families affected by his disease eventually got their first piece of good news, with the discovery of the gene responsible for Huntington's.

At the most fundamental level, we now know exactly what causes Huntington's disease. The scientific explanation is that the gene has too many repetitions of the sequence CAG, so the huntingtin protein, for which the gene is a recipe, has too many glutamine amino acid building blocks, and that makes it toxic to brain cells. If we could interrupt that simple chain of events, it would surely result in an effective treatment for Huntington's. This simple problem at the heart of Huntington's disease is also why I sometimes call it 'the most curable incurable brain disorder'. The same cannot be said for the more common neurodegenerative diseases like Alzheimer's, Parkinson's or motor neurone disease. In those conditions, only a small minority of cases have a clear genetic cause, and in the vast majority, we have no idea what triggers the premature death of neurons. The closest we can get is to look at the brain after death and see what proteins have built up, then try to develop drugs to get rid of them. In some ways this is like trying to prevent a party by designing a robot that picks up empty beer cans. Success in developing treatments for those common conditions remains frustratingly elusive, despite decades of research and billions of pounds spent.

The idea that a cure or treatment for Huntington's should follow smoothly from the discovery of its genetic basis is certainly one thing that attracted me to the field, and one reason why the Huntington's research world has more than its fair share of brilliant scientists. For the same reason, the community of people affected by Huntington's disease is intrinsically intertwined with the community of scientists trying to solve the problem. It's estimated that for every person with Huntington's disease, there are another three family members either at risk or destined to develop the disease in the future. For members of Huntington's disease families, the decision to invest time, money or effort contributing directly to scientific research is not just a tribute to the legacy of those who have succumbed, as it is in other diseases – it is also an investment in the hope of a better future for oneself or the next generation. The search for the Huntington's gene was led by Nancy Wexler and her sister Alice, who established the consortium of gene-hunters after discovering their mother had the disease. Many others have followed a similar path. After thirteen years, inevitably many of my closest friends are people I've met professionally. Some of those belong to families affected by Huntington's disease: they have the mutation themselves, or they haven't been tested, or they escaped the inheritance themselves but want to help their relatives who are sick or still at risk. So now, what started out for me as an intellectual and scientific challenge has become something more: a race against the clock, to help my friends and their families, Charlotte among them.

One of my proudest moments since I started working on Huntington's disease was in 2017 when, sitting in a wood-panelled meeting room at the headquarters of

Ionis Pharmaceuticals in San Diego, California, I saw a graph that made me weep with joy. For the first time, it showed that the drug we'd been testing since 2015, a strand of designer DNA, was doing what it was supposed to do: it was lowering production of the mutant huntingtin protein in the spinal fluid. This was unquestionably the biggest therapeutic success we'd had since the discovery of the gene in 1993. We had, in effect, a volume-control knob for the core harm that causes HD. But that was merely a numeric victory: we still had to test whether the drug – later called tominersen – would slow the progression of the disease.

Injecting 120 milligrams of tominersen into Charlotte Raven's spine in 2019 was another proud moment.

As one of our most enthusiastic clinical trial volunteers – though not our most patient patient – Charlotte would often enquire whether recruitment had begun for the phase-three trial and whether she would be in or miss out. The Gen-PEAK study started after the main, double-blinded phase-three trial, and was designed to understand how quickly the drug entered and left the body, and how quickly it started to lower huntingtin production. It had the unique advantage that everyone in Gen-PEAK would get active treatment – no placebo injections.

After Gen-PEAK was approved by the ethics committee, we held a recruitment meeting and thankfully Charlotte was at the top of the list on the basis of age, disease severity, medications, CAG repeat count and so on. She would be invited to be Gen-PEAK patient one.

The one snag was that when we had last measured her weight and height for another study, Charlotte's body mass index, or BMI, was slightly lower than the minimum requirement for the trial. Skinny is generally an advantage when it comes to lumbar puncture or insertion of an intrathecal catheter because in slender people the place we're aiming for with the needle is easier to find and hit. But this trial had been set up with a minimum BMI requirement and Charlotte, who has always been tall and thin, fell just on the wrong side of it. With my privileged, hegemonic male fingers, I duly emailed this renowned feminist thinker to tell her she had to gain weight. This was more than a little awkward. Happily, she confirmed she was willing to eat more puddings to get into the trial.

At the screening visit, prior to signing the consent form, the study doctor and patient participant read through the trial information booklet together, to ensure the volunteer has a clear idea of what will be involved and what risks they are taking. Charlotte had no trouble understanding all this, but baulked at the section – included at the behest of the ethics committee – stating that there is no direct benefit to the patient from taking part, and reminding them that the main reason to consider participating is to benefit others. 'Fuck altruism,' countered Charlotte, 'I want the bloody drug.' I had to admit, I would probably have had the same reaction – though, for the sake of getting where we needed to be, after some discussion we came to an agreement acknowledging that the overarching purpose of the trial was to contribute to the betterment of humanity, and that was generally a good thing.

Early in the trial programme, I'd started playing Beethoven's 'Pastoral Symphony' on my phone to calm the mood for tense lumbar puncture dosing sessions. I did this for Charlotte's spinal catheter insertion, too. After just a few bars, Charlotte made her opinion known. 'Will someone please turn off that fucking noise?' I didn't have any of the 1990s Madchester Indie music she preferred, so we opted for a soundtrack-free catheter insertion. Because Charlotte was the first patient in the study, I had opted to stay overnight in the clinical trial facility to personally collect the nocturnal samples. I wasn't going to volunteer to have a catheter inserted into my spine to find out what it felt like, but I could at least share some of the inconvenience Charlotte had signed up for, like being woken up at 11 p.m., 3 a.m. and 7 a.m. for spinal fluid sampling. The interrupted sleep and stress made for an exhausting week, for both of us.

The catheter went in on Monday, and I gave Charlotte her first dose of tominersen on Tuesday – one day before her fiftieth birthday. I don't think anything particularly momentous was said, but for me the ninety-second dosing window where the plunger slowly descended the barrel of the syringe and the huntingtin-lowering drug made its way into her nervous system was a brief moment to contemplate the point to which our intertwined journeys had brought us. After it was done, we hugged. Later, since Charlotte was unable to leave the hospital, I bought a passionfruit cheesecake from Waitrose and some birthday candles. Like Charlotte, I was relieved that the copious vomiting she later experienced was down to the cheesecake, not the drug.

When I heard in early 2021 that Roche had suspended dosing in the tominersen programme, because the safety committee had determined it was unlikely to be effective, it was like a punch to the guts. My nine years of work on the programme was trivial in comparison to the dashing of hope for HD families across the world. It was particularly cruel that the news came in the middle of the big coronavirus surge, so I couldn't even hug any of my colleagues or patients, and had to tell Charlotte and the others by phone of the trial's negative outcome. Our clinical research had been severely disrupted by COVID, too, so to try to help get things back to normal, I'd thrown myself vigorously into the mass-vaccination programme, at one point having personally vaccinated more people than the country of France. That's why they put my face on a vaccine bus; I haven't moved on from Huntington's – it remains my life's work. Charlotte's frustration and sense of being abandoned is entirely understandable nonetheless.

I'm still processing what it means and waiting to hear whether there is a way ahead for the drug. We will pore over the data and figure it out. Perhaps some people benefited at some dose that we can try again, or maybe we need to test it earlier in the disease when the brain is healthier. Either way, we are already trying multiple alternative approaches, including gene therapy and pills that alter the splicing of DNA. It's what the drug-hunters call a 'full pipeline'.

Tominersen was unquestionably the best drug we've tried, and the best hope for many of my patients and friends affected by HD. The huntingtin gene and its toxic protein *are* the cause of HD, and targeting them is still the most likely thing to succeed. That graph I saw in 2017 and the knowledge that we can control production of the protein cannot be taken away: they amount to what computer gamers call a 'save point'. The negative result for tominersen is a terrible blow, but at least we don't have to go all the way back to the start of the story, the gene discovery in 1993: we return to 2017 and figure out a better way to turn that success into something meaningful for people like Charlotte, Anna and John.

I don't know whether an effective treatment for Huntington's will be developed in my lifetime, or ever. I can only promise that we will keep trying.

Acknowledgements

There are many people I would like to thank for their help with this book:

I never called Susan 'Mum' but her spirit is interwoven in my past and my present, and in every conversation I have with Anna and John, which should have been witnessed by her. She would have been so proud of me and it is heart-breaking to have got this far with her as a ghost.

I still miss Murph – he was an enigmatic presence, and never less than dignified in his life or his illness. It was such an effort for him to speak when he became ill, but we cherished his good humour in the middle of this unfolding trauma. One of his last projects, unfinished at the time of his death, was a poem called 'The Last Great Whale', which has been a constant source of amusement for me, Anna and John.

This book was born from personal collaboration with Dan, my brother and the only other surviving Raven. It evolved around my kitchen table and he dressed it up well enough to be sent out into the world. No one else could have done this, as he knows me better than I know myself.

Julian Fox, a friend of my father's, has stuck around when others fell away. He used to take me to visit Murph and now comes to see me every week, so he has picked up the baton by supporting me.

Clare Alexander, my agent since the 90s, has never shied away from honest feedback even when it was hard to hear. It was her idea to combine different perspectives from me and Ed. It really means something to me that she likes this book, as she certainly isn't one for faint praise.

Alice Fisher helped me throughout the project, always able to meet the tightest deadlines with apparent ease. More than a copy-editor, she translated my feelings in the last chapter into coherent copy, as I am no longer able to type. She has also been a consistent and compassionate presence in my life.

I met Becky Seery at a writers' retreat in Sheepwash, where we had fireside chats about our work. She knows how hard it is to be a writer and always empathised. It was her idea to write the blog that allowed me to test my confidence before writing this book. Deborah Dooley, who ran the retreat and understands how to nurture creativity, kept the wine flowing and the constant technical issues with my second-hand computer in check.

Marcia Farquhar has been a sisterly support and supplier of weekly flowers and advice on men (specifically, learning to expect less from them), which has been both prudent and necessary. She read the first draft of the book and I was so happy that she liked it. She also helped with the photographs, and her husband Jem Finer corralled me into a good outfit for the photo shoot.

I was worried that, as a psychoanalyst, Stephen Grosz would make me lie on the sofa and free-associate about my dreams when what I really needed was a paternal presence and an intelligent sounding board for my ideas, personal and intellectual. But he never minded giving me advice.

Siobhan Desai, my carer and friend over the last four years, has always been available for the early-morning fags and advice sessions that have kept me sane when everything else around me was wheeling.

Finally, this book is dedicated to my children, Anna and John. They have stuck with me as allies, supporters and the loves of my life, and were uncritical readers of the book when I needed that. This book is my last will and a testament to them.